MUSIC-MAKING IN U.S. PRISONS

MUSIC-MAKING in U.S. PRISONS

Listening to Incarcerated Voices

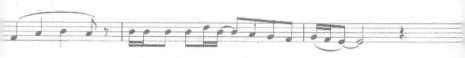

MARY L. COHEN &
STUART P. DUNCAN

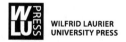

WILFRID LAURIER
UNIVERSITY PRESS

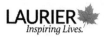

This book has been published with the help of a grant from the Canadian Federation for the Humanities and Social Sciences, through the Awards to Scholarly Publications Program, using funds provided by the Social Sciences and Humanities Research Council of Canada. Wilfrid Laurier University Press acknowledges the support of the Canada Council for the Arts for our publishing program. We acknowledge the financial support of the Government of Canada through the Canada Book Fund for our publishing activities. Funding provided by the Government of Ontario and the Ontario Arts Council. This work was supported by the Research Support Fund.

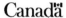 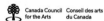

Library and Archives Canada Cataloguing in Publication

Title: Music-making in U.S. prisons : listening to incarcerated voices /
by Mary L. Cohen & Stuart P. Duncan.

Names: Cohen, Mary L., author. | Duncan, Stuart P., author.

Description: Includes bibliographical references and index.

Identifiers: Canadiana (print) 20220176892 | Canadiana (ebook) 20220176930 |
ISBN 9781771125710 (softcover) | ISBN 9781771123389 (EPUB) | ISBN 9781771124409 (PDF)

Subjects: LCSH: Music in prisons.

Classification: LCC ML3920 C678 2022 | DDC 365/.668—dc23

Cover design by John van der Woude, JVDW Designs.
Front cover image: "Jazz Band," a painting by Jason Chengrian. The musical excerpt is
from "Remember: Be Love," a song by Michael Blackwell, Sr. and Rebecca Swanson.

© 2022 Wilfrid Laurier University Press
Waterloo, Ontario, Canada
www.wlupress.wlu.ca

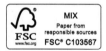

This book is printed on FSC® certified paper. It contains recycled materials and other controlled sources, is processed chlorine-free, and is manufactured using biogas energy.

Printed in Canada

Wilfrid Laurier University Press is located on the Haldimand Tract, part of the traditional territories of the Haudenosaunee, Anishinaabe, and Neutral Peoples. This land is part of the Dish with One Spoon Treaty between the Haudenosaunee and Anishnaabe Peoples and symbolizes the agreement to share, to protect our resources, and not to engage in conflict. We are grateful to the Indigenous Peoples who continue to care for and remain interconnected with this land. Through the work we publish in partnership with our authors, we seek to honour our local and larger community relationships, and to engage with the diversity of collective knowledge integral to responsible scholarly and cultural exchange.

CONTENTS

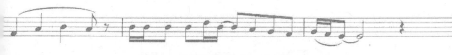

US INCARCERATION, THE PRISON INDUSTRIAL COMPLEX, AND BUILDING RELATIONSHIPS

For centuries, retributive and punitive approaches have been the norm in dealing with criminal behaviour in the United States. Problems related to prisons grew exponentially in that country in the last quarter of the twentieth century, as did those related to extended restrictions such as probation, parole, and electronic monitoring, even while the prison system was rapidly expanding. Long before these developments, federal judge James Edward Doyle (1915–87) had written about the toxicity of prisons. It was clear to him that the outcomes of prison were unbearable, and in 1972 he argued for an end to their use:

> I am persuaded that the institution of prison probably must end. In many respects it is as intolerable within the United States as was the institution of slavery, equally brutalizing to all involved, equally toxic to the social system, equally subversive of the

brotherhood of man, even more costly by some standards, and probably less rational. (Doyle 1972, 544)[1]

Between 1972 and 1976 the number of incarcerated people in the US rose 13 percent, from 250,042 to a record high of 283,268. In 1976, when incarceration rates were 88 percent lower than today's, a group of researchers and writers from the Prison Research Education Action Project led by Fay Honey Knopp, a Vermont Quaker, realizing that prisons were not solving social problems, called for their abolishment. In *Instead of Prisons: An Abolitionist Handbook* (Knopp et al. 1976), they described new responses to crime that they believed would create safer communities and ensure social and economic justice for everyone. These responses involved consideration for all survivors of crime as well as reconciliation within a caring community. They called for an end to the myth that protection, deterrence, and punishment work. We have yet to achieve that end, but we can begin to do so by paying attention to the language we use when referring to incarcerated people. The words we use infuse the actions we choose. Instead of referring to incarcerated individuals as felons, offenders, inmates, or criminals, in this book, except when we are quoting others, we purposefully adopt people-centred language such as "incarcerated individuals" or "people in custody" as a step toward changing perceptions. Given the number of wrongful convictions in the US, which Kelly Walsh and colleagues (2017) at the Urban Institute in Washington, DC, estimated at 11.6 percent, it is also clear that as a result of false testimony, false accusations, misidentification, perjury, and official misconduct, far too many people are behind bars, and that their incarceration does not necessarily signal criminal behaviour.

In a later publication, Knopp (1991, 182–83) argued that media and law enforcement portray justice in terms of a "war model," with people who commit crimes being represented as the enemy. She argues that a war model response to economic, social, political, and cultural problems has failed and will continue to do so. Crime survivors' needs, she noted, are rarely placed at the centre of legal processes, and in cases of sexual victimization, the victims are usually blamed and must prove their injuries. Also, perpetrators' needs for resocialization, re-education, and restoration are rarely considered when sentences are being handed down. She called for feminists to create a coherent and well-articulated analysis to counter war-model responses to sexual crimes. Otherwise, she argued, our society would foster an increasingly punitive and caged society (183).[2] Influenced by Knopp's project, Canadian Quakers expressed similar views in 1981:

> The prison system is both a cause and a result of violence and social injustice. Throughout history, the majority of prisoners have been the powerless and the oppressed. We are increasingly clear that the imprisonment of human beings, like their enslavement, is inherently immoral, and is as destructive to the cagers as to the caged. (Canadian Yearly Meeting of the Religious Society of Friends 1981)

Knopp's efforts did not gain much traction. Indeed, the situation got worse. At the beginning of the twenty-first century, the United States had the highest incarceration rates in the world. According to the Prison Policy Initiative, 2.3 million people were incarcerated in 1,719 state prisons (in 2012), 109 federal prisons (in 2020), 1,772 juvenile facilities (in 2016), 3,163 local jails (in 2016), 218 immigration detention centres (in 2020), and 82 facilities owned and operated by tribal authorities or the US Department of the Interior's Bureau of Indian Affairs, which include jails, youth and adult detention centres, and other justice centres (in 2020) (Sawyer and Wagner 2020; US Department of Justice 2020). People are also incarcerated in military prisons, civil commitment centres, state psychiatric hospitals, and prisons in US territories. When the Covid-19 pandemic took hold, incarceration rates dropped 15 percent to 1,215,800 in 2020 (Carson 2021).[3]

Emily Widra and Tianna Herring of the Prison Policy Initiative compared the incarceration rates of every state in the US with those in other countries and reported that thirty-four US states had higher incarceration rates than El Salvador, the country with the world's second-highest rate of incarceration (Widra and Herring 2021). Furthermore, incarceration is only part of a broader system of control that includes probation (3.6 million people) and parole (840,000 people) (Sawyer 2016). And mass incarceration has a direct impact on 4.9 million formerly incarcerated individuals, 19 million people who have been convicted of a felony, 77 million people who have a criminal record, and 113 million adults who have an immediate family member who has been incarcerated (Sawyer and Wagner 2020).

Why are these numbers so high? The four decades between 1970 and 2010 have seen a more than 700 percent increase in the incarcerated population in the US. The reasons for this are rooted in complexities that have arisen from the interactions of racial injustice, policing, sentencing, legal practices, and a dearth of programs to address addiction and mental illness. Additionally, police presence in US schools and approaches to student discipline have brought into existence a "school-to-prison pipeline," sometimes called the "school-to-prison nexus" (Meiners 2011). The latter refers to how schools are part of a web of policies, practices, and institutions that lead predominantly Black youth into prisons.[4] Disciplinary measures such as zero tolerance policies, out-of-school suspensions, expulsions, and policing of schools by resource officers have created a channel through which students—especially students of colour and students labelled with disabilities—come into direct contact with juvenile legal systems (Wilson 2014). This system relies on punishment, power, and coercive control rather than education, programming, and concern for meeting students' needs. Education professor Bettina L. Love asks, "How do you matter in a country that would rather incarcerate you than educate you?" (Love 2020).

There are currently five main types of confinement facilities in the US: local city or county jails, state prisons, federal prisons, youth facilities, and alternative facilities. Termed "remand centres" in Australia, Britain, and Canada, jails in the US are where people are incarcerated before or after adjudication, while awaiting trial if they are not granted or cannot afford bail, prior to transfer to a prison after sentencing, or when serving a sentence of under a year for a misdemeanour. Generally, sheriffs operate jails, and through consultations with judges and county attorneys, they determine how a sentence will be served—inside jail, or in-home detention with electronic monitoring. According to the Bureau of Justice Statistics, jails also temporarily house juveniles, people who are experiencing symptoms of mental illness, witnesses for courts, and people in state or federal custody because of lack of space in prisons.

People incarcerated in federal facilities have been convicted of breaking federal laws, and people serving time in state facilities have been convicted of breaking state laws. State laws differ across the US, and some crimes fall under both state and federal categories. Because each of the fifty states has its own laws and judicial policies, approaches to crime and incarceration vary widely from state to state. John Pfaff contends that we have 3,144 different criminal legal systems in the US, one for each county in the country (Pfaff 2017, 13–16).

Correctional facilities have at least four security levels: low, minimum, medium, or maximum. Two other terms frequently used are "close security" and "supermax." These terms describe security levels that are maximum and higher. The different levels denote prison authorities' perceptions of the safety risks an incarcerated individual presents. Custodial employees' evaluations, as well as reviews by counsellors or treatment facilitators, affect the security classifications of individuals. Generally, a person's path through the prison system starts at a higher level of security and eventually moves to lower levels. An individual's move from one level to another inside a prison is determined in part by their behaviour while incarcerated. Placement decisions can also be affected by favouritism as well as authorities' personal and institutional biases. Such decisions are complicated and have great consequences for all who live and work inside prison facilities.

Prison environments are detrimental not only to people who are incarcerated and their custodians but also to families and the public at large. Researchers have coined the term "correction fatigue" to describe a cluster of symptoms correctional officers can develop, which include declines in health and functioning, negative personality changes, and socially dysfunctional thinking (Denhof, Spinaris, and Morton 2014). A review of 224 studies published between 1996 and 2018 found that the prevalence of post-traumatic stress disorder in correctional officers was more than three times the national prevalence (Regehr et al. 2019). Outside the prison itself, families of people in custody face their own struggles.

The Adoption and Safe Families Act of 1997 (P.L. 105–89), while noble in its goal of improving children's safety, removed parental rights from many people in custody. This created difficulties in establishing good, safe child care and made parenting extremely challenging for people behind bars. Some of these children are placed in foster homes, with mixed results (Chipungu and Bent-Goodley 2004).[5] Family members of people in custody must deal with social, emotional, and economic stresses which are only heightened by incarceration.

The year 1997 marked an important milestone—that was the year the incarcerated population in the US passed 1.2 million. It was also the year that Drs. Angela Y. Davis, Ruth Wilson Gilmore, and others founded the group Critical Resistance (CR) with the goal of abolishing the prison industrial complex (PIC). Like Knopp's war-model interpretation of justice, the PIC broadly refers to the overlapping interests of industry and government, which together resort to policing, imprisonment, and surveillance as solutions to social, political, and economic problems. The PIC has entrenched itself in many aspects of our lives. The project of abolishing it challenges the assumption that controlling and caging people makes us safe and replaces it with the assumption that what makes communities secure is satisfaction of basic human needs for shelter, food, and freedom. CR leaders call on us to imagine new approaches that acknowledge these basic needs. In the inaugural CR conference in 1998, more than 3,500 academics, activists, restored citizens, labour leaders, policy-makers, and activists gathered to discuss the following theme: "Critical Resistance: Beyond the Prison Industrial Complex."

CR has investigated the capitalistic practices embedded in the PIC, highlighting its ability to generate profits for numerous companies. While correlation is not causation, it is telling that the rise of incarceration in the US has tracked directly with rising profits for those who provide incarceration and surveillance services, as well as for those who contract for subsidized prison labour. Private businesses accumulate capital by charging incarcerated people and their families for phone calls, electronic communications services, digital services, and food and hygiene products (i.e., those that are purchased in prison commissaries). Companies also gain from state health care contracts, transport vans, background checks, and bail bond financing; all of these strengthen the interdependent relationships between prisons and profits. In the present system, high incarceration rates and long sentences yield far greater financial rewards than the provision of meaningful rehabilitation and effective reform.

Tylek, McCleskey, and Rose (2020) of the not-for-profit organization Worth Rises report that 4,135 corporations have profited from mass surveillance and mass incarceration, including 385 publicly traded corporations and 118 investment firms. On the basis of a "harm score" they have designed to measure human rights violations, Tylek and her colleagues recommend that people not invest in ninety-five of the publicly traded corporations and sixty-one of the investment firms included in their study. These corporations include bail companies; electronic-monitoring providers; financial services; data and information systems; health care, equipment, operations, and management services; transportation and communication services; facility construction and maintenance services; food services; and prison commissaries that sell food, electronics, stamps, paper, clothing, hygiene items, health products, recreation items, and other products.

Many of the companies that fuel the PIC do so through legal monopolies and retail markets that move goods directly from warehouses to prison facilities. Having captured the prison market, these companies do not have to invest significantly in marketing to consumers, nor do they need to price their goods in competition with other suppliers. Prisoners are, quite literally, a captive market (Raher 2018). Compared to companies that operate in the non-captive market, prison suppliers enjoy sky-high profit margins. Stephen Raher estimated in 2016 that the commissary market, including government-run commissaries, brings in approximately $1.6 billion in revenues annually (Raher 2016).

Corporate mergers have further tightened this monopolistic control of the prison market across the United States. Keefe Group, founded in 1975, early in the rise of mass incarceration in the US, merged with Trinity Services Group in 2016, forming TKC Holdings. According to Raher, this merger enabled the company to collect half the total commissary revenue from the US prison market. Further analysis by Raher reveals that TKC Holdings enjoyed 42.9 percent revenue growth between 2017 and 2018, in part by reducing product quality.

Some companies have maximized their profit margins by devaluing the health and safety of those who are incarcerated. The Michigan Department of Corrections (MDOC) used private companies from 2013 to 2018 to provide food services that turned out to be unsanitary. Reports from the G. Robert Cotton Correctional Facility (part of the MDOC) described the prison food supply as infested with maggots, stored in conditions leading to mold, and containing dirt rather than actual food. Working with private companies, MDOC not only introduced unsanitary conditions but also placed the prison population—staff and incarcerated people alike—and their families at risk. In another report, when MDOC contracted with food supply company Aramark from December 2013 to 2015, it replaced its 370-state-employee workforce with lower-paid workers who smuggled drugs and contraband into prison, drank or used drugs on the job, and engaged in sexual relationships with people in custody (Egan 2015; Perkins 2018a).

In addition to these issues that compromised health, the portion sizes of food allowed under Aramark were so small that people in custody needed to purchase supplemental food from the commissary, assuming they could afford to. After Trinity merged with Keefe, the company profited from the sale of prepackaged foods in the commissary—a disincentive for the improvement of kitchen food services (Perkins 2018b). This devaluation of service was felt most acutely by incarcerated individuals who could not afford to purchase additional food. When the quality of prison-provided food deteriorates, the physical and mental health of incarcerated individuals is increasingly at risk.

The practice of building businesses upon the incarceration of other humans is problematic on several levels. It assumes that prisons are a solution to complex social problems; furthermore, as noted earlier, cost-cutting measures damage lives. Journalist Shane Bauer, who had been incarcerated in Iran for twenty-six months after he unwittingly hiked near the Iranian border while working as a freelance reporter in the Middle East, spent four months undercover working at one of the oldest privately run medium-security prisons in the US. At the time, Corrections Corporation of America (CCA) owned the facility.[6] In addition to the multiple human rights, health, and security violations within this privately run prison, Bauer (2018) describes the company's emphasis on profit over rehabilitation and re-entry, explaining how prisons in the South evolved directly from slavery. Bauer weaves historical examples of the economic and inhumane components of slavery and of post–Civil War forced labour into his own experiences as a corrections officer. As an example, he writes about Damien Coestly, who was incarcerated in Winn Correctional Center in Louisiana. Damien had filed a grievance because officers had placed him on suicide watch without consulting mental health staff. He was on suicide watch seventeen times in about forty-two months before he died by suicide. By then, he weighed only seventy-one pounds. His death occurred in a hospital, so CCA asked the DOC to grant him a "compassionate release," which it did. Because of that, CCA did not have to report his death as a suicide within its facility (161–67).

In 2015, the year that Bauer worked at Winn, CCA reported $1.8 billion in revenue, more than $3,300 per prisoner (39). CCA officially rebranded as CoreCivic in October of 2017[7] and reported $1.77 billion in revenue and a net income of $178.04 million, and had 12,875 employees (CoreCivic, Inc. 2018). Other private prison companies were finding the business of incarceration similarly lucrative. The largest private prison company, the GEO Group, had a 2017 "sales" growth of 3.9 percent, $2.26 billion in revenue, a net income of $146.24 million, and 18,512 employees (GEO Group 2018). The combined revenue of these two private prison companies in 2017 was $4.03 billion.

In 2016, Deputy Attorney General Sally Yates criticized private prisons for not offering the same level of services, safety, and security as facilities operated by the Federal Bureau of Prisons (Zapotosky and Harlan 2016). She planned, in conjunction with the US Justice Department, to phase out the use of private companies to run prisons. This goal is hard to achieve, given that the PIC is intrinsically linked to lobbyists and political agents. The GEO Group gave generously to then presidential nominee Donald Trump's campaign, and the results of the November 2016 election curtailed Yates's plans. In 2017, Attorney General Jeff Sessions reversed the 2016 Justice Department's plan to phase out private prisons. This led to significant stock price increases of 21 percent for GEO and 43 percent for CoreCivic (Gidda 2017). These same companies also contracted with the government for privately run Immigration and Customs Enforcement (ICE) detention facilities. In the first week of his presidency, Joseph Biden signed an executive order forbidding renewal of any private contracts for federal prisons, which included only eight of the 130 federal facilities.[8] That order is largely symbolic; it indicates a federal effort to change, but deciding not to renew private contracts does not advance a shift toward implementing newer, healing forms of justice, nor does it address the racist roots of policing and prisons in the US, or the massive profits gained from companies who service prisons.

Professor Elizabeth Hinton, a specialist in African and African American Studies at Harvard, argues that federal programs intended to decrease crime have often been punitive and inequitable. She points to the Law Enforcement Assistance Administration (LEAA), started in 1965 and disbanded in 1982, which provided federal money for 80,000 crime-control policing projects. That funding expanded local supervision in urban communities with low-income populations, and as a result, more youth of colour were arrested. According to Hinton, efforts by both Democratic and Republican presidents, while aimed at improving the public good, have in fact contributed to the US's position as the world leader in incarceration, as well as a prison population disproportionately composed of black and brown people (Hinton 2016).[9] Erica Meiners, a Professor of Education and Women and Gender Studies at Northeastern Illinois University, has described the US mass incarceration crisis as "targeted criminalization" (Meiners 2016, 2).

There remains a pervasive trend in the US toward dehumanizing incarcerated people and ignoring the realities of incarceration. Michael Santos describes this punitive emphasis as socially counterproductive in his book *Inside: Life Behind Bars in America*:

> If the end goal is to warehouse human beings, then the American prison system is a costly but effective design. However, if the goal is to prepare people to live as law-abiding, contributing citizens, then objective data suggest that our prison system is a stellar example of failure, ripe for reconsideration. (Santos 2006, xxiii)

At the time he wrote those words, Santos had served more than twenty years in US federal prisons. One of his most compelling observations was about correctional officers' harsh treatment of people in custody. He wrote that the prison staff "make it clear that they have the power to lock us away, to separate us from our family members for longer periods. To them, we're nothing but registration numbers" (243). Wilbert Rideau, who spent forty-four years incarcerated in the Louisiana State Penitentiary at Angola, made a similar observation about how staff treated the people in their custody.[10] According to him, the biggest challenge in prison is "the way you are assaulted psychologically and emotionally, the way in which you are robbed of any dignity as a human being" (Rideau 2010, 338). During his time in prison, he spent more than three years in solitary confinement and eight years in a one-man cell on death row.

US prisons routinely use solitary confinement as a security protocol, a practice that has been cited as cruel and unusual punishment. UN Special Rapporteur on torture Juan E. Méndez (2011) noted that solitary confinement should only be used in exceptional circumstances and for as short a time as possible; he also maintained that solitary confinement of more than fifteen days should be completely prohibited. Such objections to solitary confinement are grounded in common-sense awareness of the social nature of humanity. Humans, as a species, live in groups and communities, and our fundamental need to connect with others makes solitary confinement a highly unnatural human experience. The use of solitary confinement in prisons leads to outcomes such as occupational and psychological hazards for correctional staff, as well as to disruption of incarcerated individuals' sleep cycles owing to a lack of exposure to natural sunlight and the unpredictable cacophony of sounds such as jangling keys, distressed voices reverberating off cement walls, and clanking metal doors. Solitary confinement is also two to three times more expensive than housing a prisoner in the general population.

Solitary confinement is a highly undesirable condition that offends against the human rights of those who must endure it. Yet Sharon Shalev, a research associate at the University of Oxford Faculty of Law, reports that prison officers and administrators frequently resort to it, completely disregarding human rights guidelines. The negative impact of solitary confinement on an individual's health and well-being is magnified when solitude is imposed without a clear time limit and on people with poor social adjustment and/or prior mental health problems—conditions that afflict many incarcerated individuals in the US. The use of solitary confinement as punishment often results in anxiety, depression, anger, cognitive disturbances, perceptual distortions, paranoia, and psychosis; it also has negative physiological effects such as cardiovascular and gastrointestinal disorders, joint pain, eyesight deterioration, migraine headaches, and profound fatigue. Shalev (2011, 175) argues that the use of solitary confinement in supermax facilities, where those in custody are on permanent lockdown, is inhumane and in direct "violation of human rights law instruments to which the United States is signatory." Despite such caveats, an estimated 80,000 people in US prisons are confined in solitary confinement today (Solitary Watch n.d.). This punitive strategy is used more in the US than in any other country in the world and more than in any other country in history (Shourd 2016, viii).

The negative psychological effects of solitary confinement on an individual's well-being are especially severe for youth. In "Scarred by Solitude," published in a collection of essays by people who have experienced solitary confinement in prison, Enceno Macy (Casella et al. 2016, 123), who moved to the Pacific Northwest upon release from prison, described his experiences in solitary. First, he spent time in solitary confinement in a youth facility at age thirteen for forgetting to ask permission to talk, being too loud, or using bad language. Then, at the age of fifteen, he was sent to an adult prison, where he spent fifteen years in and out of solitary confinement. He noted that his experience "made me feel as though I wasn't meant for this world. I still feel that way to this day—like I don't fit." Ten years after his release, Macy still experiences panic attacks so severe that he requires antidepressants for PTSD, feels lonely, and finds it difficult to trust others.

Solitary confinement is an obvious human rights abuse encountered in US prisons, but there are others, one of which is excessive sentences. Although there is little evidence that long sentences have a deterrence effect (Nagin 2013, 231), prison sentences in the US continue to be longer than in many other countries. The average US sentence of 63 months (Bonczar 2010) compares with 4 months in Canada, 10.1 months in Finland, and 13 months in England and Wales, while in Germany, the majority (92%) of sentences are under 24 months (JPI 2011). In the US, mandatory minimum sentencing laws require the judge to set a determined length of time for people convicted of state and federal crimes, and this has disproportionately affected minorities. Additionally, as of 2016 more than 200,000 people were serving life or virtual life sentences, and more than two-thirds of those individuals were people of colour (Nellis 2021).[11]

In 1976 the death penalty was reinstated in the US in *Gregg v. Georgia*, making the United States one of a handful of countries, including China, Iran, Saudi Arabia, Iraq, and Egypt, and the only country in the Americas, with capital punishment as a legal penalty. This stands in stark contrast to a large number of countries, some of which are not based on democratic governance, that are abolishing capital punishment.[12] Since 1976, 1,533 people have been executed in thirty-five states, and others have been executed by the federal government (Death Penalty Information Center n.d.). In 2020, during the Trump administration, the US put to death more people who were in federal custody than in the previous fifty-seven years.[13]

These extreme sentencing practices violate Rule Four of the Nelson Mandela Rules, adopted by the UN General Assembly on December 17, 2015. Those rules delineate the UN Standard Minimum Rules for the Treatment of Prisoners. Rule 4 states the following:

1. The purposes of a sentence of imprisonment or similar measures deprivative of a person's liberty are primarily to

protect society against crime and to reduce recidivism. Those purposes can be achieved only if the period of imprisonment is used to ensure, so far as possible, the reintegration of such persons into society upon release so that they can lead a law-abiding and self-supporting life.

2. To this end, prison administrations and other competent authorities should offer education, vocational training and work, as well as other forms of assistance that are appropriate and available, including those of a remedial, moral, spiritual, social and health- and sports-based nature. All such programmes, activities and services should be delivered in line with the individual treatment needs of prisoners. (UN General Assembly 2015)

US adversarial legal systems also contrast sharply with long-standing Native American dispute resolution methods that promote community harmony and encourage perpetrators to be accountable and take responsibility for their actions (Johnson 2007). Navajo people conceptualize "law" differently than the Anglo-European tradition. The Navajo word for "law" is *beehaz'aanii*, meaning something fundamental and absolute that has existed from the beginning of time. It is a source of a healthy, meaningful life. Rather than a "vertical" system of justice that relies on power and hierarchies, Navajo justice is "horizontal," described best as a circle that symbolizes unity, oneness, with no beginning or end, where every person in the circle looks to the same centre as a focus. This sense of "solidarity," although difficult to translate from Navajo to English, includes concepts of reconciliation with community, family, nature, and all reality, as a path to restoring good relations with others and with oneself (Yazzie 1994).

Rather than following the Nelson Mandela rules or the Navajo justice approach, the US has developed a massive punitive machinery.

In 1968, concern for lack of critical thinking about penal policy, crime, human dignity, and diversity prompted a group of sociologists from the UK to gather at the Institute of Criminology at Cambridge, where they attempted to close the gap between theory and practice. They formed the National Deviancy Conference[14] involving academics, a prisoners' union, radical lawyers, and radical social workers, to mark the birth of critical criminology. Three key thinkers in this new branch of criminology, Ian Taylor, Paul Walton, and Jock Young, were especially critical of "the systemic nature of criminalization under capitalism" (Mintz 1974, 43). They proposed that crime be understood as "an authentic form of consciousness" (Mintz 1974, 39). Accordingly, critical criminology considers the onset of crime and the essence of justice within social structures and status inequalities, including socio-economic discrepancies that intersect with race and with policies that explicitly or implicitly discriminate against Blacks.

Black scholars, activists, and artists in the US have long written about the inequities brought about by systemic racism.[15] Perhaps the best-known Black peacemaker, Martin Luther King, Jr. (1929–68), during periods of incarceration in Georgia jails, wrote sermons about forgiveness and loving one's enemies. In his "Love in Action" sermon, he described society's slowness to forgive and defined capital punishment as "society's final assertion that it will not forgive" (King 1963, 57). He called for an awareness of the errors of US history, such as the 1857 Dred Scott decision, segregationist practices, and the myth of inferior and superior races, all of which have fed into present-day mass incarceration. Foreshadowing ideas of peacemaking criminology, in his "Loving Your Enemies" sermon King (1963) conveyed the need to develop and maintain the capacity to forgive (73), asserting that goodness exists within those who have hurt others (74–76) and warning that hate injures the hater (79). He assigned his listeners the challenge of love and forgiveness: "While abhorring segregation, we shall love the segregationist. This is the only way to create the beloved community" (85). Such ideas prepared the ground for goals of this book and are foundational to restorative justice and its application to critical and peacemaking criminology.

Peacemaking criminology emerged as a branch of critical criminology in the late 1970s and early 1980s. This school of thought was founded by Indiana University Professor of Criminal Justice Hal Pepinsky and University of Wisconsin sociologist Richard Quinney, who proposed realistic and constructive ways to think about troublesome human interactions. As a response to violence and the harm it causes, peacemaking criminology acknowledges that violence and peacemaking are both processes that can simultaneously expand and contract. Pepinsky (2013) believed that responsiveness is the opposite of violence, so he wanted to find ways to increase the extent and improve the quality of people's ability to respond to one another in human relationships. Much of his thinking on this developed while he was studying on a Fulbright Fellowship in Norway, translating his thoughts into Norwegian, and engaging in dialogue with renowned sociologist Nils Christie (1928–2015). Pepinsky's interest in the concept he called "responsiveness" originated in his Norwegian translation of three English words: responsibility, liability, and accountability (320), and was influenced by his studies with Christie.

Christie was a teenager when the Nazis occupied Norway. In his master's thesis, he sought to understand how Norwegian and German camp guards experienced Yugoslavian prisoners of war, 70 percent of whom were killed or died from sickness and starvation during the Second World War. Christie's investigation uncovered two categories of guards. One subscribed to the official German position that the prisoners of war were so awful that they had to be deported from Central Europe in order to keep the peace. Christie described these guards as killers and maltreaters. The other group, who did not kill or maltreat the Yugoslavians, were distinguishable from the first primarily by their greater proximity to the Yugoslavians. The non-killers saw photos of the families of the men in their custody, while the killers generally did not

(Snare 1975). A central principle of Christie's thinking was that the level of punitive treatment varies according to how much one knows about the person who is to be punished (Wagner 2015).

Building on Christie's principle, Pepinsky's notion of responsiveness considers the process of developing trust through hearing stories, noticing feelings, and adapting responses to the goal of establishing safety and extending social care through honest interactions. In response to Christie's conclusion that time with others can build trust and relieve fear, Pepinsky (2013, 337) asserted that "violence is driven by fear, peacemaking by love and compassion." Although Pepinsky acknowledged that people are generally more practised at conquering and dominating others than at peacemaking with themselves or others, he believed that peacemaking had the potential to actually transform rather than temporarily suppress violence. Denying the existence of a politically neutral understanding of "criminality" or "crime," Pepinsky described peacemaking as a political process that cannot be imposed, but instead must unfold within the situational context of the people involved (Pepinsky 2013, 335–37).

Accountability and forgiveness play a central role in the more healing approaches to justice that Christie and Pepinsky envisioned. New Hampshire Representative Renny Cushing is someone who has developed an awareness of these issues. In 1988, his father, Robert G. Cushing, Sr. (1926–2006) was murdered by two shotgun blasts through the family's screen door. Cushing reported:

> Before my father's murder I had evolved a set of values that included a respect for life and an opposition to the death penalty. For me to change my beliefs because my father was murdered would only give more power to his killers, for they would then take not only his life but also his main legacy to me: the values he instilled. The same is true for society. If we let murderers turn us to murder, we give them too much power. They succeed in

bringing us to their way of thinking and acting, and we become what we say we abhor. (Murder Victims' Families for Human Rights n.d.)

Cushing helped abolish the death penalty in New Hampshire with the acknowledgement and support of crime survivors. In 2004, he and a group of victims' family members founded "Murder Victims' Families for Human Rights," and Cushing was behind House Bill 455, which repealed the death penalty in New Hampshire in 2019. Other exemplary grassroots healing approaches that seek to enact positive change are Danielle Sered's (2019) Common Justice model of survivor-centred and racially equitable responses to violence that do not rely on incarceration (Common Justice n.d.) and the UN *Handbook of Basic Principles and Promising Practices on Alternatives to Imprisonment* (Smit 2007).

Solitary confinement is a non-responsive reaction to criminal behaviour; so is the sheer isolation that prison inflicts. Imprisonment in the US tends to sever family and community relationships and impose dominating, punitive relationships. Yet from birth, humans rely on one another to survive, so in many ways we are hardwired to connect with one another. According to social neuroscientist Matthew Lieberman (2013, 5), the neural overlap between physical and social pain confirms our profound need for social connection. Also according to him, our need to connect with others is more basic than our need for food or shelter. When incarcerated, human individuals seek connections with others, and the types of connections they make—positive or negative— impact their behaviours. Similarly, their family members, including the more than 5 million US children burdened by the emotional weight of incarcerated parents, need meaningful connections with their loved ones behind bars; and those behind bars need to feel connected with a positive community, ideally including their family members.[16]

In place of solitary confinement, long and drawn-out sentences, punitive psychological and physical harm to incarcerated people, and pervasive punishment after release from prison, we advocate in this book for opportunities to listen to incarcerated voices, work collaboratively with people impacted by justice systems, and share emotional expressions in new ways to create spaces for personal and social transformations. Stephen John Hartnett, a prison educator and Professor of Communications at the University of Colorado Denver, suggests that to move toward social change, there must be a "fundamental change in consciousness" (2011, 8) rooted in a pedagogy of empowerment and hope.

This fundamental change in consciousness will require a long-term social and cultural transformation that takes multiple approaches. Bryan Stevenson, founder of the Equal Justice Initiative and author of *Just Mercy: A Story of Justice and Redemption* (2014), maintains that "mercy is most empowering, liberating, and transformative when it is directed at the undeserving. The people who haven't earned it, who haven't even sought it, are the most meaningful recipients of our compassion" (314). Stevenson's insight resonates with our goals in this book. Like him, we seek to foster the growth of compassion in our understanding and treatment of ourselves and others, starting with a deeper social awareness of the harmful aspects of prisons.

The American historian Robin D.G. Kelley (2020) argues that to rework the PIC, we will need to continually interrogate every form of oppression. In their book *Prison by Any Other Name* (2020), Maya Schenwar of the not-for-profit news organization Truthout and journalist Victoria Law (2020) contend that popular prison reforms are themselves forms of oppression. They call for a social welfare system that would provide for children's and families' needs and for grassroots support and healing and that would transform systems of justice and community accountability. Above all, they call for building relationships within neighbourhoods, something that will take time and is "not as automatic as dialing 911" (235).

To build relationships and the ability to be responsive, as Pepinsky recommended, we can apply the ideas of Bryan Stevenson (2014), who, like Nils Christie, has suggested that proximity can motivate members of a society to realize one another's needs. Bringing together incarcerated individuals and people from outside the prison, including members of the wider community, offers opportunities for new relationships and perspectives to develop. But not just any interaction will work. Engagement with the potential to inspire change must be purposeful, creative, expressive, and capable of motivating both personal and social transformation. We envision musical leaders taking such a direct, purposeful, and transformative approach to music-making in prisons with clear intentions of building responsivity that creates caring communities.

Arts programming in prisons allows participants and audiences to create pathways toward new relationships, imagine approaches to decarceration (reducing the number of people in custody) and excarceration (establishing alternatives to prisons such as mediation centres), build social responsibility, and move toward reconciliation. Over the past decade, arts programming in prison contexts has steadily expanded nationwide. One driver of this growth was a series of conferences hosted by the William James Association and California Lawyers for the Arts between 2015 and 2019 that brought together formerly incarcerated people, artists, activists, and scholars to share practices and to network (CLA n.d.). The Justice Arts Coalition (JAC) grew out of these meetings and now provides collaborative spaces for reimagining justice through the arts.[17] Through these and other joint ventures, arts facilitators in collaboration with incarcerated artists have witnessed many negative impacts of incarceration, developed mutually meaningful relationships, and observed transformative changes among participants.

The impact of JAC artists on US criminal legal systems has yet to be measured, but some positive signs have emerged. In tandem with the increase in arts programming, visual and theatrical arts programs in US prisons are attracting scholarly attention. In 2020, James Weldon Johnson, a Professor of Media, Culture, and Communication at NYU as well as a 2021 MacArthur Fellow, and Nicole R. Fleetwood published *Marking Time: Art in the Age of Mass Incarceration* (2020), which contains images of work by incarcerated artists and explores the creation of visual art in confinement. Fleetwood's analysis includes reflections on photographs she has received over the years from her cousin Allen, who was sentenced to life in prison when he was eighteen, as well as descriptions of art made in solitary confinement. The volume includes ninety-six illustrations of visual art created in custody and invites a deeply critical look at the racially formed structures of incarceration, calling on readers to imagine and create "a world without human caging" (Fleetwood 2020, 263). Fleetwood points to the capacity of artmaking to "disrupt the mandate of prison" (25). She seeks to cultivate relationships between people in custody and the broader public but warns that artmaking in prisons can be a tool for further racial discrimination regarding who is allowed to participate.

Different than visual arts, theatre is a performance-based arts practice that relies heavily on working together, thereby offering opportunities to build relationships based on collaborative artmaking. In her examination of drama practices in prisons across ten countries, Ashley Lucas, Associate Professor of Theatre and Drama and Director of the Prison Creative Arts Project at the University of Michigan, contends that theatre created in prisons provides a space for group interactions and human connections but that the unequal power dynamics in institutions complicate these programs (2011). Nevertheless, she argues that theatre can be a means to disrupt the redemption narrative, which problematically assumes that people's criminal behaviour should define them for the rest of their lives.

Mariame Kaba, founder and director of Project NIA, is an abolitionist organizer who aims to end youth incarceration. She emphasizes the vital role that artists can play in disrupting patterns and making us feel and think differently. Art, creativity, and PIC abolition work together, she maintains, because this type of abolitionist thinking is about "imagining a new way" (Madden, Leeds, and Carmichael 2020). Key points for transforming society, according to Kaba (2021, 4), include being in intentional relationships with one another, imagining ourselves differently, and experimenting with and building "collective responsibility."

Throughout this introduction we have highlighted the need to completely reimagine the PIC. At the centre of our call for action is an understanding of the harms caused by the PIC and the need for effective communication, collaboration, attentive listening to others' stories, and motivation to build caring relationships. These changes are starting through arts programming in prisons, and it is now time to expand these practices with clear, constructive, and transformative intentions.

Like theatrical performance, music-making requires cooperation in the name of collective responsibility. In the process of rehearsing, people in musical ensembles work to establish a common pulse, listen for consonance and dissonance, experience shared lyrical messages, benefit from the physiological experiences of singing, and collectively encounter emotional expression and social action. Research and practice both suggest there is strong potential for building relationships through innovative music education programming in prisons that uses collaboration and co-creation to build proximity and responsivity (Cohen 2012a; Swanson and Cohen forthcoming).

Music-making with others, especially with people from different social and ethnic backgrounds, offers opportunities to connect with one another, to build a broadened sense of family and community, and to create more compassion and care. When incarcerated and non-incarcerated people interact musically, their shared experience helps them notice how much they have in common, as illustrated by the case studies described throughout this book. A change of hearts and minds through an awareness of common humanity is a vital step in making consequential changes to punitive systems.

Songwriting and choral singing, when facilitated effectively, provide a means for people behind bars to express emotions, thus empowering their unheard voices. People outside of prison who listen to or sing alongside people inside prison can create spaces to connect meaningfully and broaden their sense of our common humanity (Cohen 2019b; de Quadros 2019). Neutral or negative outcomes are possible for musical participants if they do not feel capable of succeeding, if they feel judged, or if the musical experience does not resonate with them. Conversely, in group singing facilitated with integrity, individual voices weave into a full communal voice, allowing people behind bars to feel more normal. From the perspective of an incarcerated singer in the Oakdale Community Choir comprised of incarcerated or inside singers and people from the community or outside singers, founded by Mary Cohen, a co-author of this book: "In regard to our choir community, I have always felt warmly welcomed and accepted by everyone. It is a unique community of insiders and outsiders. For the hours we spend together each week, those differences are cast aside, and we are not insiders and outsiders. We are choir members, a community, a family."[18]

An inside singer in the Oakdale Choir, Kenneth Bailey, wrote the lyrics of the song "One More Look." Kenneth's opening phrase "Don't cast me in the mold you forged without knowing my intentions" and his message in the chorus about "a better way to build a future from what's here today" together highlight the importance of seeking more information about ourselves and others. The phrase "I'll lay down my father's sword, that's made with all his imperfections. And I'll listen to the words you speak as we search for a new direction" can be interpreted as challenging the listener to seek more information about others and ourselves rather than making assumptions, and to be curious, not judgmental.[19]

"One More Look"
(Spring 2012, Lyrics by Kenneth Bailey, Music by Mary Cohen)

Don't cast me in the mold you forged
without knowing my intentions.

Lay aside your weak assumptions,
so we can harvest our convictions.
Examine all the differences,
That should have never been created.
Then from us through our children,
All these lies can be deflated.

CHORUS
One more look, and tell me what you see,
Just one more look,
Perhaps we'll both believe
That there's a better way
To build a future from what's here today:
And there's a second chance
Just one look away;
A second chance, one look away.

I'll show you who I am inside
And please accept this gift I'm giving.
If we can't renew what once we had
How can we say that we are living?
I'll lay down my father's sword
That's made with all his imperfections
And I'll listen to the words you speak
As we search for a new direction.

Interpreting Kenneth's words, we read that in order to move in a new direction, people need to listen and seek a deeper awareness of their own and others' intentions, laying aside assumptions and examining differences and their origins. Music-making and listening to the voices of people in prison together create social bridges and transformative thinking. After attending an Oakdale Choir concert in the prison gym, a board-certified music therapist, Gloria Hartley, reflected on her experience: "I once heard someone describe 'stigma' as distance, and I think, where stigma exists, the space that exists in that distance is easily filled with fear, assumptions, stereotypes, caricatures, and judgements. The Oakdale Community Choir concert closed that distance, both literally (this is the first time I have ever been inside a prison) and figuratively—to create instead a space where connection happens." Given the complex issues that surround criminal legal systems, we may need, as Ruth Wilson Gilmore (2022) suggests, to "change everything." The systems that need changing are indeed multiple and complex—schools, policing, legal systems, behaviours, and attitudes.

We can learn a great deal from perspectives outside of the US (de Quadros 2019). In this regard, Mariame Kaba argues that PIC abolition is both an internationalist project and an anti-capitalist one (Madden, Leeds, and Carmichael 2020). This book, however, focuses on US practices, partly because it is a first step toward growing awareness of music-making in prisons and partly because of the contextual aspects of human rights issues in the US. Grounded in the experiences of past practices of music-making in US prisons and recent programs from music educators from around the US, our book examines the successes and challenges faced by those who are facilitating programs, acknowledges the potential negative experiences and outcomes of music programs in prisons, distills the pedagogical aspects that foster success, explores ethical and power structure issues related to facilitating musical communities in prison contexts, addresses challenges for music-makers in prisons, and provides suggestions for how musical communities can be seeds for transformative changes in the broken criminal legal systems. We must boldly imagine what is possible to promote transformative changes, collaborate with and learn from others directly impacted by the systems, listen to these voices, build leaders in change-making, and explore new ways that music-making can contribute to these processes.

Using personal experiences, accounts from fellow teachers, and critical examinations of past programs as a starting point, we want to encourage widespread engagement with musical learning and its capacity to help shift the US away from a carceral state. Police, prisons, probation, parole, and electronic monitoring might be set aside in favour of methods that make us less reliant on punitive approaches, thus strengthening our ability to truly listen to others, mutually support one another's needs, and build caring communities. Scholarship on prison issues has been attracting a growing audience—particularly regarding the roots of racial and economic inequities, suggestions for decarceration, and many approaches toward abolition—and we believe it is important to encourage the synthesis of past and current practices of music education in prisons to further radical transformation from punishment-focused, racially inequitable systems into completely new ways to co-create caring communities.[20]

Punitive responses to crime only dig deeper into people's wounds rather than creating an environment for healing. We highlight the history and present practices of "us and them" approaches to criminal punishment systems and contrast how music educators and activists have the potential to invoke a "we" mentality. Unfortunately, certain musical practices in society have enabled various "us and them" attitudes. For example, some individuals think that people either can or cannot sing and so do not realize that singing is a *learned* skill. The idea that someone cannot sing comes from an evaluative, performance model. This type of attitude is highly problematic when we try to establish group singing in prisons. Some incarcerated individuals think they cannot join a choir because they cannot sing and may not be willing to try. Some administrators do not understand that all people have the potential to learn to sing and can benefit from the group singing experience as they are learning to sing. When a primary emphasis shifts from an evaluative model to an inclusionary and experiential model, the social and relational aspects of music-making become the primary goals and the experience feels inclusive—a vital need for all, especially for people who are incarcerated.

In addition to exploring how an inclusionary model of music-making can work in prisons, this book provides a starting point for people who participate in musical learning to recognize possibilities for purposeful innovation in their approaches to teaching and learning, to apply insights from historical and contemporary research about music education in prisons, and to consider how music educators can work toward abolition, even within their K–16 classrooms. This potential to invoke a "we" mentality, which we argue for in this book, is even stronger when people facilitating music-making in prison contexts and in schools create pedagogical spaces for relationship-building and proximity with individuals and cultures from a variety of life backgrounds. These points are especially important for music educators, for about half of the music education faculty members who completed a survey about their perspectives on social justice defined the concept with "difference-blind" language—equal opportunities for all without awareness of differences related to historical oppression through colonialism, patriarchy, capitalism, heterosexism, and white supremacy (Salvador and Kelly-McHale 2017, 13–14). The examination of music-making in prisons we offer in this book provides insight into how social justice perspectives can be incorporated into music teaching.

We explore the complexity and possibilities of creating space for survivors of crime to feel a part of this "we" mentality and suggest that arts and music practices can be a path toward healing (Lederach 2005). Music educators have begun to develop more inclusive pedagogies, and the time is now ripe for a deeper consideration of the roles of music education to (a) broaden awareness of our common humanity, (b) implement innovative creative programming, and (c) support all young learners using strength-based teaching and empowering learning approaches. We realize that music-making in prisons will not solve all the problems we have presented in this chapter, but we aim to introduce the reader to research, practice, and pedagogies that have the potential to bring people into relationship with one another in ways that inspire personal and social growth and public awareness of the need to imagine positive, sustainable changes.

Our book demonstrates the power and impact of music-making within US prisons, how it can play a role in the transformative overhaul that countless experts have been calling for, and how it enables people, both inside and outside prison walls, to encounter a sense of healing justice.[21] Music-making inspires new identities, meaningful relationships, and courageous self-expression; it gives voice to those who have not had a voice. Humans are imperfect, and we continue to make mistakes, but how we, as individuals and as a society, unpack the many complex human challenges in our lives and respond to broken relationships can allow us to co-create caring communities. The potential for bold approaches in music education is ripe for building positive social connections and transforming society from a culture of revenge into a culture of caring.

CHAPTER 1

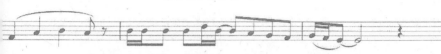

WHY MUSIC-MAKING
IN PRISONS?

Music-making builds relationships among people both inside and outside prison walls and has the potential to create change on the level of the individual as well as broader changes in society's perception of incarceration. However, achieving these things is by no means guaranteed. Unpacking the opportunities and challenges these goals present is a core purpose of this book. We posit that music-making involving incarcerated and non-incarcerated musicians provides a platform for amplifying their voices. Music-making can reveal the harmful aspects of the prison industrial complex (PIC), thus broadening society's awareness of the changes needed for the US to end its infatuation with incarceration. Ultimately, music-making can inspire innovative pedagogical approaches that lead toward transformative changes for incarcerated individuals, their families, custodial staff, and society.

None of the proposals we put forward will be easy to implement, and they have their own unforeseen consequences. Over the course of this book, we will unpack and explore these complexities by first understanding how past music programs may have succeeded and then by considering first-hand accounts from current practitioners. We will reflect on past and current programs through several theoretical lenses including restorative practices, transformational theories, desistance theory, critical criminology, and peacebuilding. For centuries, music-making has been a part of prison life, organized by people in custody. An example is singing or playing instruments for worship. While there is value in that form of music-making, we will be focusing on secular music-making.

Our understanding of music-making is rooted in Christopher Small's (1927–2011) concept of musicking. Small (1998, 9) treated the word "music" as a verb. "To music," according to him, is "to take part, in any capacity, in a musical performance, whether by performing, by listening, by rehearsing or practicing, by providing material for performance (what is called composing), or by dancing." According to Small, the relationships between sounds and people are the most important aspect of musicking. The essential meaning of music, for Small, rests "in action, in what people do" (8). Everyone present in a musical activity, including rehearsals and performances, is involved in musicking. Small suggests that we ask, *"What does it mean when this performance (of this work) takes place at this time, in this place, with these participants?"* (10, italics in original). We need to understand both the how and the why behind any musicking experience.

Once incarcerated, people are referred to by a number and their last name, and, depending on the institution where they reside, they have limited opportunities to make their own decisions. Musicking for people in custody can provide agency in subtle yet potentially meaningful ways. Small's concept of musicking is the conceptual framework for my (Cohen's) theory of interactional choral singing pedagogy in prison contexts. I theorize that when facilitated effectively, choral musicking in prison contexts can foster measurable personal and social growth (Cohen 2007a, 292–95). Contemporary research and practice has tested this theory, and anyone interested in this topic is encouraged to study these investigations and further this research.[1]

Before we examine how music-making builds relationships, let us consider how it can foster an incarcerated individual's relationship with oneself, particularly when their identity has been stripped away by harmful systems. In the process, they can develop a fuller aware-ness of their own feelings as well as build self-efficacy. Mick Jones, an incarcerated or "inside" Oakdale singer, was a member of the combined outside–inside choir that performed "Dear Younger Me," written by Oakdale Choir inside singer Perry Miller. Perry had responded to a prompt to write advice to yourself as a younger person. Mick shared the following deeply personal reflection prior to the song's premiere:

> I am twenty years old, but I have the life experiences, injuries, of someone twice my age. If I were to write my response to the prompt to "Dear Younger Me," I wonder, should I tell myself to not follow the inconsistent ways my mother modelled? Should I warn myself about the abuse of being beaten by whatever was at hand? Should I warn myself of being adopted into a well-mean-ing but seriously misguided family? Should I mention the many heartbreaks and lost loved ones that I would have? All in all, I would probably tell myself to follow my heart more.

Through singing Perry's song and considering how he would respond to the prompt to reflect upon his younger self, Mick examined his own broken and difficult past. He demonstrated the courage and vulnerability it takes to express such deep, personal experiences twice: to an audience of his peers in the prison, and to about eighty-five out-side guests, along with prison staff and administrators.

Another inside-Oakdale singer, Rick Trevors, composed the lyrics to "Inside the Fences," set to music by Mary Cohen. The title is a play on the multiple meanings of two words: inside and fences. *Inside* represents both an individual's interior emotional landscape and a physical space. Looking at the lyrics as a whole, his words "The world seems so angry. It's hard to forgive us. That's why the fences are so high" might suggest a lack of forgiveness and responsivity from society as among the obstacles that block connectivity between society and imprisoned people. His lyrical expressions also seem deeply rooted in his personal religious beliefs and experiences:

> Lord, we have been looking and trying to find the way outside.
> You alone understand the things we are hiding from
>   ourselves and all the others.
> We say we love, we say we love.
> You alone must show us how to change, from the inside.
> *From the inside, inside, from the inside.*

1. The world seems so angry. It's hard to forgive us
    That's why the fences are so high.
    The cars are pulling up out front.
    The ones that we love are trying to come inside.
    Not knowing the hurt that goes on
    Behind the fences.

2. Lord, I finally listened and heard you calling my name.
    I have come a long way in that calling you gave.
    Your words are hiding in my heart and on my tongue
          every day.
    How can I open up and feel what's inside?
    To let the healing begin,
    For that's the only way to change

> *From the inside. From the inside. Inside, from the inside, from*
> *the inside.*

3. I'm doing slow laps on a short track, watching time go by
   I'm doing slow laps on a short track
   Watching the world go by
   As we work to change
   From the inside, the inside, from the inside.

Rick's lyrics, "Your words are hiding in my heart and on my tongue every day. How can I open up and feel what's inside?," suggest a yearning for a deeper self-awareness and a connection to his emotions. Such expression behind bars is difficult given how people in custody are separated from the outside world and how formidable the obstacles or "fences" are that surround their feelings.

In my efforts to create a collaborative process for setting his lyrics to music, after I (Cohen) set Rick's lyrics to a four-part choral harmony, we used the Liz Lerman Critical Response Process to discuss the lyrics and musical setting (Borstel and Lerman 2003).[2] Through this process the songwriters discussed how difficult visits were— some preferred to not have any visits so they would not be reminded of how separate they were from society. Rick shared how the musical setting was too complex for what he had envisioned. In retrospect, I (Cohen) should have paid far closer attention to his compositional vision. From my perspective, the song we created included important messages for the outside singers and audience members to hear. Singing, the physical experience of using breath, voice, and musicality, offered a space for the emotional expression of his first-hand knowledge of life behind bars. Audiences who heard his words gained a glimpse of how difficult it must be for a person whose interactions with the world are stopped, as he spends his days "doing slow laps on a short track, watching time go by."

Prison systems are designed to prevent social interaction, to minimize individual expression, and to control through security measures. The physical restrictions of incarceration disrupt established relationships, both familial and community. This in turn prevents the incarcerated individual from developing essential social connections that would aid in the transition back into a community outside of prison. If we agree that it is important that, post-incarceration, a person be given every chance to succeed, to be able to contribute to society in meaningful rather than harmful ways, then the prohibition on social connection and friendship combined with the deprivation of individuality sets them up for failure.

Laya Silber, senior teacher and choral director at the Bar-Ilan University in Israel, led a choral program in a maximum-security women's facility in Israel. She reported that when her university choir came into the facility for a choir-to-choir songfest, it was a highlight of their choral program. The university choir performed for the women and sang with the women for two songs that had four- to five-part harmonies. The incarcerated singers previously had only performed two-part harmonies. One of the incarcerated singers wrote: "It was as if we were inside each others' voices...we are a little bit on the outside, they are a little on the inside with us" (Silber 2005, 268). In addition to the musical connections evident through singing together, Silber reported choir members' increased social sensitivity through improved listening skills and eye contact. They curbed their aggression through breathing and the use of head voice, strengthened their trust in others, developed a sense of group support through harmonic back-up, and learned to delay gratification through long-term preparation for a performance. The choral singing rehearsals and performance laid the foundations for community associations, a sense of feeling cared for, and empowerment through a humanizing and normalizing activity—all so different from daily prison life. The fact that outside volunteers chose to enter the prison facility to sing with incarcerated individuals built a sense of trust and sent a message to them that they were worthy.

During the first season of the Oakdale Choir in Iowa in 2009, John Marcus, an incarcerated Oakdale singer, wrote:

> When I first heard of the choir being put together I was excited and kind of nervous all at the same time. I wasn't sure what to expect. Would I be good enough to sing with others? Would they be afraid of me since I'm an inmate? ...The first night our guests showed up I felt ready for the challenge. As we walked about and talked to each other, I knew at that moment I would be accepted graciously. The thoughts of being in prison went away and I felt relaxed. (OCC Oakdale Community Choir Newsletter 2009)

Being together in the context of a choir softened this man's earlier fears of being around people from outside the prison. All had gathered for the purpose of singing together, and the interpersonal interactions, both informal and formal, created opportunities for new social connections.

Another prison choir member, Steven Walker, wrote:

> The choir here at Oakdale provides a great opportunity for personal interaction. It is also a great forum for conveying values and exchanging perspectives. For some of the inmates here, it is the only personal interaction possible, other than with guards and other inmates. This lack of personal contact is not healthy, either socially, emotionally, or psychologically. Thanks to all who seek to breach the wall that isolation builds. (OCC Oakdale Community Choir Newsletter 2011)

Bringing together people from outside the prison with people who are incarcerated creates a social connection for people who have had few interactions other than with people within the institution. Those interactions provide openings for sharing thoughts and discussing ideas, something this person found highly meaningful.

Inside singer David Frazier explained that he wrote the song "My Family" for his personal family, but he has since grasped that the song is also for his choir family: "The choir has done so much for me, given me hope and light, and they are a part of my family too." When someone considers the people in their musical ensemble their family, they have developed a sense of group responsibility and communal identity with the other people in the ensemble, as David's lyrics about unity and togetherness seem to indicate:

"My Family"

There is a road, on it we travel, all alone, and lost.
There is a light, that we foresee,
That light is my family,
We may never know the cost of the road we have crossed,
Carry on, and maybe someday, we all can say:

CHORUS
My family, we are one.
My family, together.
My family, look what we've done.
My family forever.

Disconnection from family is a particularly difficult fact of imprisonment. One of the many challenges families face is maintaining positive connections with one another despite this physical disconnection. The long and strenuous experience of "doing time" can be assuaged to some extent through musical learning and performing activities in prisons. Music-making can bridge separations in unique ways (Cohen et al. 2021).

In Kansas, the men in custody who sing with the East Hill Singers (EHS) leave the minimum-security unit of Lansing Correctional Facility to perform with outside volunteers in public venues. Family members tend to find concert attendance rewarding because performances are celebratory events and include enjoyable music and opportunities to see loved ones excel. Nieces and nephews under eighteen do not qualify for visits in most US prisons, but they can attend EHS concerts. Forrest Moret's first EHS concert was on his mother's sixty-fifth birthday on January 8, 2006. Forrest's older brother Bill, angry with Forrest's drug use, self-sabotage, and apathy, vowed not to visit Forrest in prison and did not answer any of his brother's letters. However, he decided to travel to Blessed Sacrament Church in Kansas City, Kansas, along with his sister Leslie, his dad Fred, his mom, Sandra, and Forrest's eleven-year-old son. A full hour before the concert, the family reunited, an opportunity that would not have come about had the choral concert not taken place in a public venue (Kavanaugh 2006).

In Oakdale Prison, children under eighteen have long been barred from the prison for Oakdale Choir concerts, but Warden Jim McKinney decided it was important for the children of inside singers to watch their fathers perform. After not seeing her father for five years, Kevin Jones's seventeen-year-old daughter, Melissa, came to a concert. Outside choir members took Melissa for ice cream after the event. Inside singer Trevor Johnson's three children—nine, eleven, and thirteen years old— attended an Oakdale concert in the prison gym and heard their father recite a heartfelt introduction he had written to Sam Cooke's song, "A Change Is Gonna Come":

> I identify emotionally with Sam Cooke's "A Change is Gonna Come." There has been pain and tragedy in my life and for a long time it felt too hard to keep going. But I kept going. When I was knocked down, I got back up. Nothing was changing in my life because I wasn't changing. Even with setbacks I am making progress and change is happening a little at a time. We changed one set of lyrics in this song. Notice the difference between the original, "brother help me please, but he winds up knocking

me back down on, on my knees." What we sing today, "Brother help me please, but it winds up not just me back down on, on my knees." Hurtful behaviour hurts the person being hurt, and the hurter.

Trevor's personal reflection resonates with points that many prison scholars have argued. It is not just the people who are incarcerated who are hurt by punitive practices. The depth of the harm is much greater and broader than most people realize. Trauma affects perpetrators, crime survivors, and family members in ways unique to each situation. The stigma of a parent in prison is difficult for a child to navigate. However, when a child sees their parent proudly perform and they experience the audience members' warm response to their incarcerated parent, a new narrative of success and skills develops, potentially relieving them of their shame and embarrassment. Music-making is an especially effective path toward meaningful social connections.

Family members of inside singers have received professional recordings from Oakdale Choir concerts.[3] These recordings allow family members to listen to their loved one performing with the choir even if they cannot travel to the prison to attend the concerts in person. They can also share these recordings with friends and listen to the performances in between visits to the prison and during the Covid-19 pandemic (when they have not been allowed to visit in person). These recordings contribute to family members' sense of pride, care, and gratitude for their incarcerated loved ones and allow outside singers and other members of society to listen to incarcerated voices (Douglas 2019).[4]

Original songs about loved ones provide a conduit for expressing meaningful personal connections that may be difficult to make through phone conversations, electronic mail,[5] or short visits (Cohen 2012a; Silber 2005). One inside singer in the Oakdale Choir, George Smith, composed "A Song for Howard" for his son. Howard was unable to attend the concert where it was performed and had in fact dropped out of high school. Soon after George was released from prison, he got out his guitar and started singing the song while his son was nearby playing a video game. Howard stopped playing the game, realizing that the song was about him. The informal sharing of his original song opened an hour-long conversation between father and son. George convinced his son to go back to high school, and he helped him with his studies. Howard was the first of his six children to graduate from high school. George hosted the graduation party at his new home, and "it was truly a blessing I'll never forget." When he played "A Song for Howard" at the graduation party, there were "tears in many eyes," including his.

Beyond individual self-reflection, there is also a strong need for connection, for proximity or direct connections with others in order to understand their stories and make meaningful changes in systems of criminal punishment (Stevenson 2014). When people interact face to face, speaking to one another and spending time together, they develop deeper understandings of one another. Choral singing and music education programs can be powerful tools for creating such proximity, especially when a choir brings incarcerated individuals and community members together as peers, be it as performers or audience members.

For example, Jennifer Fish, a volunteer with the Inside Out Reentry Community, an Iowa City not-for-profit that provides support for people released from prison, noted that her passion for volunteering with that organization strengthened after she attended an Oakdale Choir concert. The experience deepened her compassion for the challenges incarcerated individuals face. She described how the concert experience was "beyond words"—"when your heart and soul are drawn in, as mine were, words are too limited to fully capture what's experienced." She described how she held back tears during the first thirty minutes of the concert, how it was her first visit inside a prison, and how she would have "rather been there than any place in the world." Her primary comment related to an original song, "I Pray for You," about an incarcerated individual's separation from his four children:

> I was most struck and touched by the unshakable story of the inside member who has four children, whom his sister kept him informed about. His strength and resolve to find what he could do, pray, for each of them, continually, and selflessly, was a testimony of faith, grace, and the things unseen. (Jennifer Fish, personal communication)

The theme of this concert was "Look on the Bright Side," and Fish noted that not only did it achieve that goal, but it was "a genuine experience of our connectivity as humans, and a humbling of the soul. Unspeakable gifts." Fish's experience of physically being inside the prison, listening to incarcerated choir members share their personal family stories, and hearing their voices perform together helps us see how music-making in prisons can bring about connections between humans, an important step toward healing and functioning well and so different from punitive responses to crime.

Maya Schenwar and Victoria Law contend that cycles of inequality continue in society because we have not yet done the necessary personal transformative work to create substantial change (Schenwar and Law 2020). That transformative work must be done at both personal and social levels. With respect to social awareness of inequality and to personal challenges that can impact incarceration, another original song, titled "That Childhood of Ours," written by an inside member of the Oakdale Prison Choir, provides opportunities for awareness of and reflection on cycles of inequality. Bill Hildebrand grew up in an abusive family, the youngest of more than six children. His parents were alcoholics, and his father beat Bill and his siblings. It was hard for him to express this song, but he was encouraged by a friend to write it and share it, for others could relate to the difficulties expressed in it:

Never had money, Mom and Dad drank it all. All in our beds
our empty stomachs would growl. Monday to Sunday they
never were sober. We were ashamed to bring anyone over.

Was beat black and blue by my own father's hand. Next day
"What happened to you?" He would demand. They'd drink
in their bed and fall asleep in the tub. Dear old Dad used his
fist like a Billy club.

Mom tried to fight back sometimes with all her might. On
those few days when her mind was mostly right. But our dad
was too big with too strong an arm. Mom never won never
escaped without harm.

From the Bloody Bucket to the Coney Island Bar, got
plenty to drink without going too far. Returned home with
a friend and a sack of food. Didn't even bother to wake their
starving brood.

We had plenty of reasons to hate them both. Plenty of reasons
for crying cussing oaths. But all we kids ever had, all we kids
ever had, all we kids ever had, was an undying love for our
mom and our dad.

It was difficult for the choir members to learn and sing Bill's song,
and equally difficult for the audience from outside the prison to hear
about Bill's abusive childhood. We performed the song in a concert
themed "Community of Caring" because the last line of the song
expresses the deep love Bill and his siblings had for their parents, even
though they were abused at their parents' hands. The performance of
"That Childhood of Ours" provided audience members an opportunity to consider the difficulties of Bill's childhood from sixty years ago,

allowing a very real personal understanding of one man who was living behind bars (Cohen 2019a, 144).

Although contemporary research about music-making in prisons is not extensive, outcomes consistently indicate that through music-making, incarcerated individuals can achieve personal growth. Through this means of self-expression, they improve their focus, develop a sense of group responsibility, and strengthen their self-esteem and their sense of worth and competence (Cohen 2012a; Palidofsky and Stolbach 2012). Music for them can be a "sanctuary" where they can improve their lives and futures and relieve their stress, but also experience difficult feelings such as regret, pain, and loss (Doxat-Pratt 2018, 165–67, 174, 181). Through music-making, people in custody can experience social growth—improved family relationships, more positive attitudes toward others, a strengthened ability to get along with others, and new friends (Cohen and Palidofsky 2013). Research also suggests that music-making in prisons broadens outsiders' perspectives of people in prison, a necessary step toward supporting returning citizens and to stretching society's imagination when it comes to considering alternatives to prisons and new healing approaches to justice (Cohen 2019b; Messerschmidt 2017).

A multilayered approach allows people in custody to develop their dignity and work to dismantle the harmful aspects of the PIC, and music-making can be one facet of that approach. Given how new music-making is in contemporary carceral systems, and the complexities of prison contexts, musical leaders need to innovate to make positive progress. We can also learn by exploring how music educators attended to teaching in prisons prior to the rise of mass incarceration.

Despite the complex challenges posed by US prison practices and the punitive nature of prison management, innovative music educators have long been teaching incarcerated individuals and creating caring communities through musical learning and musical ensembles. These communities have provided bridges between the outside and inside worlds. For decades, music-making in prisons has shown its potential to create communities of care, deepen awareness of the need to overhaul US criminal legal systems, and inspire people both inside and outside to take more positive, healing approaches to justice. Today's carceral systems do not address the root causes of social ills; rather, they perpetuate them. Issues of economic inequality and structural and institutional racism, as well as the faulty assumption that policing and prisons make society safer, have limited citizens' and community leaders' imaginations about possible new pathways. Arts and music programs in prisons can generate shifts toward new approaches rooted in healing justice. Next, we investigate past programming, pairing that discussion with the wisdom of abolitionist thinking to provide inspiration for what might be possible.

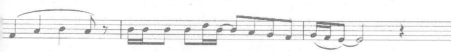

CHAPTER 2

"MIGHT IS NOT ALWAYS RIGHT"

Historical Reflections on Music-Making in US Prisons

*B*efore the rise of mass incarceration, US prison administrators often supported music-making activities. Such activities were seen as a valuable and effective support mechanism for incarcerated individuals and as a meaningful way to connect people inside and outside of prisons. Take, for example, the programming of Willem van de Wall (1887–1953), who served as a director on the use of music in prisons and other institutions in New York State. He argued that traditional jails and prisons bred "an evil spirit in men" and sent them into the world "trained and fully prepared to perpetuate and intensify criminality and suffering in society" (van de Wall 1924, 16). What was needed was "communal unity" and "a feeling of social well-being" (18).[1] Music is not a cure-all, but it offers new possibilities that emphasize love. One man in custody, upon leaving a musical performance inside a 1920s prison, reportedly said, "We have feelings too. The people on the outside forget that, and we forget it too. But this music brought it out and back" (28).

Van de Wall argued that when a society hates people in custody, it reaps what it sows: "bitter aversion, continued hostility, detestation, abhorrence, more crime, more misery, more losses, and an endless chain of ignominious offences" (19). Given how punitive approaches have intensified since van de Wall wrote those words, a heightened need exists for envisioning a different society based on mutual aid and co-operation rather than policing and imprisonment (Kaba 2021, 17).

Additional insight into the role music historically played in US prisons is provided by Moritz Liepmann (1869–1928), a professor of criminology at the University of Hamburg, who toured, inspected, and studied US prisons in the autumn of 1926. He was critical of many aspects of the prisons he visited; however, he was complementary of van de Wall's use of music in prisons, mental hospitals, and training schools:[2]

> It is this function of music that gives it its educational value. Releasing and discharging stored up emotion as it does, it saves the inmates of an institution from that hardening of the heart, that intensification of hatred and longing for revenge, that accumulation of feelings of inferiority and unsatisfied, suppressed desires—in short, from all those destructive psychic conditions which constitute the most serious problem that educational work in prisons and training schools is called upon to solve. Music appeases and releases; it provides opportunity for self-expression, which Americans rightly recognize as a valuable substitute for repression, with its unwholesome consequences. There can be no question that such a freeing of emotional energy can be made a highly important factor in the maintenance of discipline and in the achievement of a

harmonious mental atmosphere favorable to good teamwork. (Liepmann 1928, 53)

Van de Wall's and Liepmann's observations invite deeper investigation into past practices and prison administrators' efforts to provide music-making opportunities for incarcerated populations.

Van de Wall and Liepmann are just two examples of historical accounts of music-making in US prisons. Further research has revealed a considerable number of additional accounts.[3] The first part of this chapter considers the broader survey-like examinations of music-making happening in prisons from the 1930s to the 1960s, drawing upon the work of seven researchers, who collectively suggest that the US used music-making in prisons holistically and viewed it as a valuable endeavour. The second part of this chapter focuses on several individual programs from the early 1900s to the 1960s and continues to consider the "why?" as it begins to answer the "how?" in response to our primary points from Chapter 1: that music-making provides a means for personal and social growth, and that increased societal awareness of our common humanity is needed to overhaul broken systems. This reflective analysis of past programming, and of current desistance theory, allows us to reimagine possible roles of music-making in prisons in society today.

Vetold Sporny (1914–2002), was a music supervisor at the Pennsylvania Training School in Morganza, a strict reform-type school, where he taught youth choral singing. His singers were under the age of twenty-one; they had been convicted of crimes and lived in cottages on the campus. In the early 1940s, Sporny (1941) researched the extent of music education opportunities in prisons for the purpose of suggesting what types of music experiences prisons might work in prisons. Through his survey, he received responses from sixty-nine institutions across twenty-four states. He established that music was required at all prisons that contained academic schools and was optional at 84 percent of the facilities (5–6). Music instructors involved in these programs had a wide range of experience; half were graduates of accredited schools but had no training to teach in institutions.[4]

He concluded that prisons should establish music-making activities based on the following order of preference: community singing, choirs and glee clubs, band, orchestra, instrumental ensembles, and music appreciation. It is interesting that Sporny prioritized vocal groups over instrumental and other forms of musical engagement. He concluded that music education supported participants' emotional expression, developed their self-knowledge, released tension, improved concentration, increased self-discipline, and acted as a socializing agent (45). One reason why music-making had more value in prisons than other forms of learning was that musicians' progress occurred because of their own ambition and efforts (12–13). Eighty-three percent of music teachers reported that people in custody enjoyed community singing enthusiastically, and Sporny strongly encouraged it as one means for the entire population to gather as a community: "No other fine art can duplicate this effect with such great number of inmates" (54).

Many of Sporny's findings are applicable today in advocating for music-making in prisons, especially its capacity to facilitate self-expression, social bonding, well-being, and motivation for learning. Thirty-five percent of his study's respondents had music ensembles that performed publicly outside the institution, anywhere from three to thirteen appearances per year. Most of the teachers favoured these public performances, offering reasons similar to those we described in Chapter 1—public performances are a strong incentive, motivation is increased, music-making inspires dignity and confidence, and musical performances and recordings can connect the public with people in prison (39–40).

A few years after Sporny, in 1951, Raymond George Hodson surveyed prison educators for his music education master's thesis at the University of Denver. He, like Sporny, wanted to compare prison music education programs across different states, but he broadened his inquiry to thirty-four states and a fifteen-year window, 1934 to 1951.[5] His survey indicated that those programs offered music appreciation, harmony, and theory classes as well as bands, glee clubs, and orchestras. Of particular interest to our study is how his respondents told him that incarcerated musicians often interacted with audiences outside the prison space. For example, he noted that men's vocal ensembles from prisons in Birmingham and Montgomery, Alabama, were broadcast on radio shows each Saturday morning (Hodson 1951, 86). Additionally, prisons in at least seven states invited outside musical groups to perform in their facilities.[6] Hodson concluded that more time should be given to promote incarcerated people's musical expressions on local radio stations and that the proceeds from public concerts should go toward supporting musicians while they were in prison or after they were released (86).

Around the same time as Hodson, in 1952, Anthony Apicella surveyed seventy institutions in nine northeastern states (Connecticut, Maine, Massachusetts, New Hampshire, New York, New Jersey, Pennsylvania, Rhode Island, and Vermont) for his master's thesis at Boston University. Like Sporny and Hodson, he wanted to establish whether prisons offered music programs and, if so, what types.[7] Fifty-eight prisons responded. The majority had religious choirs; 25 reported that bands were part of their programming (Apicella 1952, 58–59); 14 had dance orchestras; 8 had concert orchestras; 24 offered instrumental instruction (84).

Apicella reported, similar to Hodson, that a wide variety of institutions used music programs as a bridge between those inside prisons and those outside them. Bands performed for ceremonies inside and outside the prisons, including graduations, patriotic events, theatrical performances, sporting events, parades, and fairs (60). Apicella's study suggested that bands in male prisons helped build community within the prison population and contributed to a positive self-identity. Also, prison band members contributed "to the enjoyment, to the discipline, and to the morale of the inmate population" (84). Band membership allowed men in custody to belong to an honoured organization, wear attractive uniforms, and travel outside the institution. Such experiences seemed to encourage identity-building, yet some prison administrators had chosen to eliminate music activities, thinking that they interfered with work programs and that it was not feasible to offer them at night (86). Apicella concluded that some directors and wardens were concerned mainly about the profits from their prison workshops, which was why they eliminated music activities (88).

In 1956, Donald J. Landreville added to the growing body of research by studying how state prisons used music in the US Northwest and in six federal prisons. He compared these music programs with activities in the Montana State Prison.[8] Musical activities included vocal instruction, choirs for church services, talent shows, and ensembles such as choruses, orchestras, bands, and dance orchestras (9). He found that the main goal of more progressive administrations during the 1950s was to rehabilitate, that wardens advocated for the use of music in rehabilitation efforts, and that music personnel enjoyed "enthusiastic support" (34). He observed that this approach differed from past methods, in which men "were placed in custody in miserable surroundings and forgotten" (Landreville 1956, 8).

Most surprising about Landreville's report is how varied the leadership of these musical activities was. Some programs had a full-time paid music director or part-time director, but most instructors were either incarcerated individuals or custodial officers with no teaching certification. For example, Landreville reported that two men in custody in Leavenworth Federal Penitentiary had successfully proposed a music appreciation class in 1949. These men, whose names were Stone and Leonard, created a 222-page comprehensive course textbook, borrowed twenty records from Chaplain Otto Lang, and started the class with sixty-five men. In the first two years of the program, more than 800 men attended classes, the library grew to 1,700 records, and new electronic equipment was acquired (66–69).

Landreville suggested that music in prisons could be used for five purposes: (a) to develop professional musicianship skills (i.e., professional musicians should continue to perform and serve as teachers), (b) to provide activities to occupy idle time, (c) to improve problematic behaviours, (d) to address social educational needs, and (e) to encourage recreation (3–4).[9] He also reported the need for more music therapists to be employed in prisons.

Landreville found that Montana State Prison personnel used the band program as a reward system. Some of the men had no prior music experience before they were assigned to the band, which was considered a full-time assignment (28–29). If they broke a prison rule and were written up, they were reassigned to other positions in the prison. One attempted escape twice, another had six write-ups, and another shifted between periods of good behaviour and disciplinary infractions. The band appeared to provide opportunities for them to build self-discipline. This reduced the number of disturbances, although the administrators at times had to offer repeated second chances for the men to try again.

Sporny, Hodson, and Apicella all surveyed various groupings of states, often by region. William J. Littell's research offers a significantly broader overview of music activities across the entire US in the mid-twentieth century. In his masters' thesis at the University of Kansas in 1961, Littell set out to assess the potential interest in music therapy programs in prisons. He collected survey responses from institutions listed in the American Correctional Association directory that had a population of fifty or more (Littell 1961).[10] These institutions included state and federal prisons as well as "penitentiaries, reformatories, training and industrial schools, juvenile detention homes, forestry camps, state prison farms, prison camps, and reception centers" (17).[11] Respondents indicated that the purposes of music in prisons included recreation, rehabilitation, avocational training, control of behaviour, and vocational training.[12] Remarkably, eighty-seven institutions (40.2%) reported that their musical groups left the prison grounds for performances or as spectators. Furthermore, 156 (79.2%) of the respondents noted the value of music programs in prisons with respect to recreation and rehabilitation (22–23).[13]

In solicited responses, one person indicated that the best aspect of music programs in prisons "is the wonderful atmosphere it creates" (54). Another wrote that when the band played for mess lines, tensions were reduced. Another indicated their music program helped incarcerated individuals learn an avocation and develop teamwork skills and self-control, besides providing opportunities for creative expression (50). Some respondents were quite enthusiastic, one of them noting that "we think we haven't even scratched the surface in this work and see an almost unlimited potential in benefits derived from a learning of better work habits and attitudes" (51). A number of respondents noted how difficult it was to employ music directors due to the limited number of applicants and the financial costs.

Other researchers besides graduate students were examining the impact of music in prisons. In a book published in 1955 about music in recreation, sociologist and musician Max Kaplan (1911–98) sent twenty-two questionnaires to administrators in state and federal penitentiaries. Twelve of thirteen who replied reported that they provided organized musical activities. These facilities were in California, Georgia, Idaho, Illinois, Maine, New Jersey, Kansas, Mississippi, and Texas. There was a wide range in terms of how long these programs had existed— between three months and "always" (Kaplan 1955, 46). Besides demonstrating the prevalence of music programs across the US, which was also evident in the surveys by Sporny, Hodson, and Apicella, Kaplan's project identified five objectives of these music programs: rehabilitation, education, entertainment, better relations with society, and contributions to special occasions (46).

Sporny, Hodson, Apicella, and Kaplan established that at mid-century, music programs were widespread in prisons across the US. Their surveys identified a variety of musical experiences, which were led by various staff and incarcerated individuals. Many of the reports noted music's powerful rehabilitative potential. Importantly, many programs offered opportunities to establish connections between incarcerated individuals and the public, whether through radio performances, public attendance at concerts in prisons, or incarcerated ensembles leaving the prison to provide music in public spaces. Furthermore, music-making provides opportunities for people in custody to express their emotions, and this reduces tensions and builds self-knowledge, concentration, and self-discipline. Incarcerated participants grow musically through their own learning and agency when rehearsing and performing, including for the public.

The support for music programming in mid-twentieth-century prisons was reflected in the 1954 *Manual of Correctional Standards* produced by the American Correctional Association (ACA), the overarching prison association for the U.S. That manual compared music to other educational experiences:

> Music is probably the cultural field most easily developed in an institution. Under a competent full-time musical director it can be raised above the usual mediocre level of institutional music and can become a cultural as well as a recreational and morale-building activity. (303)[14]

The ACA emphasized the value of high-quality instructors: "The importance of well trained recreational and physical education directors, arts and crafts instructors, and music teachers cannot be overestimated. The personnel provided is even more important than the equipment" (90). This emphasis on music-making and quality instructors went beyond construing music as simply a form of recreation; it could become a core component of educational programs as well as a cultural touchstone. This emphasis on creating spaces for music education programs aligned closely with the organization's desire to support incarcerated individuals' individual agency and their learning to connect positively and meaningfully with others (409).[15]

Two years after the ACA manual was published, in 1956, the 86th Annual Congress of Correction met in Los Angeles. It attracted 1,300 delegates from forty-eight states, the District of Columbia, Alaska, Hawaii, Canada, China, England, Iran, Japan, and Puerto Rico and had the goal of documenting the need to create opportunities for freedom for incarcerated individuals:

> *Minds can be freed only when we create the opportunities for free-dom.* We do not rehabilitate—we do not reform—we do not convert. We have the solemn obligation to create the opportunity for minds to be free to find themselves and the truths by which they can live in harmony with their fellow men. (*American Journal of Correction* 1956, 11, italics in original)

One way people in prison can develop a sense of "freedom" is by connecting with the public; another is by building a sense of normalcy through social links with society. Reed Cozart (1956b), a pardon attorney working for the Department of Justice in Washington, DC, called for people from outside prison to develop and promote socializing programs for people in prison, including music clubs (24), joint participation in performances, and presentations by high school bands and church choirs (1956a, 27). The mid-twentieth-century philosophy of correction, as encapsulated by these groups, contrasts strikingly with today's US prison management, which focuses on suppressing individual agency, and limits at best and negates at worst, the interactions for those outside to participate and gain from interacting with incarcerated people. The positive impact described in the summaries of these mid-century research studies came from the relationships fostered among musicians and between performers and audience members. Connections with people in the community through music-making occurred naturally as incarcerated individuals entrained to a common pulse, sang or played in the same key centre, shared lyrical messages, experienced physiological aspects of singing or playing, and participated together in emotional, physical, and social activities. Factors like these all contributed to normalizing experiences that may bring a sense of freedom. Such connections are vital for people living in prisons because the effects of institutional living involve dependence on institutional structures; hypervigilance and distrust of others; social withdrawal and isolation; and feelings of diminished self-worth (Haney 2001). By deepening our awareness of past programming, we can consider how music-making can be one tool for building proximity with people in custody and growing our imaginations to create supportive environments.

Beyond these academically framed surveys, there are a number of resources that allow us to develop a more detailed picture of individual music-making programs and to investigate how, and in what ways, music programs began and the successes and challenges they have encountered. The following publications, dating back to 1907, indicate how music education has long served as a conduit for personal and social growth for people in custody and built connections between society and incarcerated populations.

In 1907, James C. Sanders (1866–1922), a music educator and cornet player, became warden of the Iowa State Penitentiary in Fort Madison. A former band director in Corwith, Iowa, professional baseball player, and umpire, he was known for saying, "Might is not always right" and "The majority is not always just and fair." He made numerous changes at Fort Madison. For example, he initiated the honour system, and guards no longer carried clubs. He outlawed beatings and solitary confinement, added barbershop and bathing facilities in the prison, and abolished the rule that men's clothing had to be the traditional striped uniform; instead, they dressed in "tailor-made suits, laundered shirts, and polished shoes" (Mullenbach 2015). On Saturday afternoons, men with no infractions could play basketball and baseball. Rather than guards bringing food into cells, the men ate in a dining room and listened to an orchestra comprised of twelve to sixteen incarcerated individuals who had purchased their own instruments with money they had earned in prison jobs.

Sanders started the orchestra with only two men from the prison population (*Le Mars Semi-Weekly Sentinel* 1909). Before they were incarcerated, one of them played cornet, and the other played violin. Shortly after, a pianist and clarinetist joined. The small ensemble rehearsed daily after they had finished their prison jobs. Meanwhile, Sanders began a glee club, initially with twenty men. He "drilled and drilled, coatless, sleeves rolled up, perspiring, late in the evenings" (2). After a few rehearsals, to the surprise of the men, he announced, "To-morrow before the noon meal in the dining room we make our initial appearance." The next day the choir performed a sacred selection for around 450 men in custody, who stood with bowed heads. That was the start of daily live musical performances during each noon meal.

Burgess Wilson Garrett, a member of the State Board of Parole, gave a glowing endorsement of Sanders' program:

> The men take immense interest in the musical organizations and there is a genuine rivalry to get into them. It conduces to good discipline and adds something of the outer life to the confinement which these men are enduring. You would not think, ordinarily, that a man confined in a penitentiary would want to sing or could sing from his heart, but they seem to be able to do it … The influence of the music and other things of that sort is excellent. (Garrett 1908)

Sanders's vision for a more rehabilitative model within the prison paired well with his background as a music educator. As Garrett noted, his efforts to bring men together to play instruments and learn how to sing and perform as a group motivated them to earn the privilege of participating and thereby create a connection to life outside prison.

In the Waupun Correctional Institution in Wisconsin, starting in 1908, Chaplain Reverend Sylvester J. Dowling (1870–1964) organized a prison brass band. The band had around thirty men, who rehearsed daily, played at meals, and performed for the local community.[16] Within two years, they had performed at fifteen different events both inside and outside the prison. Warden Henry Town (1861–1932) reported: "The influence of the musical organizations, the band, orchestra and choir, as well as the entertainments provided, has been very manifest. To the men it means light and cheer, and drives away the darker shadows of Prison life, so productive to melancholy, disobedience, revolt and punishment" (Cary 1910, 184–85). These musical ensembles continued into the 1920s. The Monday evening weekly performances that were held in the summer of 1924 on the front lawn of the prison provided community leisure activities and connections between the musicians in the ensemble and the people of Waupun and the surrounding area. Warden Oscar Lee noted that they planned to continue the following summer. He thought the band should grow in size and quality and have a full-time music instructor (Lee 1924, 3).

In the Nebraska State Penitentiary, William T. Fenton (1873–1939) served as warden from 1913 until 1934. Like Warden Lee in Wisconsin and Warden Sanders in Iowa, he made improvements in the prison, increasing officers' wages, stopping the rule of silence at meals, allowing men to wear civilian suits for Sunday chapel, and treating the men in custody with respect. He supported the start of instrumental ensembles in the prison. Just as at Fort Madison in Iowa, the band performed daily at lunch and during Sunday prison chapel services. Also, just as in Iowa and Wisconsin, the Nebraska musical groups provided a bridge between people inside and outside prison walls. Members of the public came into the penitentiary on Christmas night to watch the men in custody perform.

The music programs provided a space for men to work toward self-improvement. One incarcerated musician had a particularly interesting journey: Antonio Ciarletta, who had served ten years in the Nebraska Penitentiary, learned to play several instruments while incarcerated, including cornet and trumpet; he also conducted the orchestra. A few days before the 1924 Christmas performance, he received commutation from the Nebraska State Pardon Board. On the day he was released, he went to the capitol to express his gratitude to Secretary of State Pool and Governor Bryan for the chance to remake his life and be home with his family for the holiday (*Lincoln Nebraska Star* 1924). With Antonio's departure, another incarcerated individual, Louis Chobar, replaced him as prison orchestra director for the Christmas performance. Louis had worked hard to build his skills and create this opportunity. He had saved a year of earnings, bought a saxophone, and practised in the chapel daily with the warden's approval. At night he silently practised his fingering (*Lincoln Nebraska Evening Journal* 1929). These anecdotes indicate that incarcerated individuals were motivated to save money to purchase instruments, to build technical and artistic skills, and to work collaboratively in order to perform for others—all examples of how music-making in prison builds self-efficacy, agency, and teamwork skills.

According to historian Mike Brubaker (2014), in addition to Christmas concerts, other prison concerts were open to the public inside the Nebraska State Penitentiary while Fenton was warden, including benefit concerts for the Salvation Army and for regional disaster relief. As a precaution against escapes, the men in custody who appeared on stage did not interact with the audience, but sometimes people from the public performed for the imprisoned men. One such performance was a chorus of schoolchildren from Lincoln, Nebraska. The inclusion of youth in public/prison interactions demonstrates a very different approach from today's: one that is open and welcoming and that fosters a positive attitude toward people who are incarcerated. Warden Fenton used these performances to support his request that the prison infrastructure be expanded to support performing arts. Specifically, he wanted—and got—a new auditorium with seating for

1,300 people and a 30-foot-wide by 26-foot-deep stage. The incarcerated men, along with staff, administrators, and community leaders, put on an annual Thanksgiving show called "The Shutin's Frolic." The event was promoted in regional newspapers. The show took place every year, but 1928 was particularly important. Seven hundred-fifty people attended the show, which was assisted by Herbert Yenre, who took charge of production (*Lincoln* NE *Star* 1928). The money from performances like these helped maintain the prison orchestra and provided funds for other recreation activities (*Lincoln* NE *Star* 1928). These regular musical performances served as a public relations tool for prison administrators. They also suggest there was a much more fluid relationship between people in the community and people in prison, compared to contemporary times.

Clinton T. Duffy (1898–1982), an outspoken opponent of the death penalty, was warden at San Quentin State Prison in California from 1940 to 1952. He accomplished many reforms at that facility, one of which was improving an existing band that eventually played at noon meals and on occasional evenings, with the live performances broadcast through the prison radio network.[17] Duffy described a Sunday afternoon in 1940 when he listened to the performance of the incarcerated musicians, wearing grey and black prison uniforms and playing "as though the parole board had just turned them down." With the help of Ted Stanich, a guard with a professional music background, he went through the files of the incarcerated men to compile a list of musicians who could play everything from a military march to a boogie. Then Stanich and Duffy rustled up some old instruments, including a piano, saxophones, and fiddles. They recruited John Hendricks, a former army bandmaster and walking encyclopedia of music who was serving a life sentence. He had been spared the death penalty and showed his gratitude by keeping a spotless behaviour record. Duffy asked John if he could create an orchestra that would play what the men wanted to hear, attract outsiders, and "chase the blues away" from prison life.

Duffy explained the rehearsal process and initial performance of the newly revitalized orchestra in San Quentin:

> John coaxed, threatened, and cussed those musicians at rehearsals far into the night, a prison Toscanini who was determined to show that murderers, thugs, and thieves can also have music in their hearts and perhaps play as well as most orchestras outside. I could hardly believe my eyes sometimes, watching certain gangsters and tough guys meekly taking John's caustic rebukes, but they had respect for his musicianship and were anxious to please. John's first jazz concert in the mess hall nearly shook the girders out of the roof, and a stranger might have thought it was a riot. The waiters took up the beat with their big metal spoons, plates were banged on the table tops and men stomped their feet on the concrete floor. There was such an upsurge in morale inside those ancient walls after the first few concerts that I decided to have the orchestra at the noon meal more often, and sometimes there was an extra performance at night which went into the cells via the newly installed prison radio network. All the inmates were proud of their hard-working band, and that pride was shown in their conduct and their work. Before long, various carefully selected lodges, clubs, and groups of peace officers from nearby towns were invited to hear the band, and word soon spread around about the new spirit in the big house by the bay. (Duffy and Jennings 1968, 235–36)

In addition to the band, a thirty-man glee club led by an incarcerated musician rehearsed with the orchestra. To four different San Francisco stations, Duffy pitched the idea for a radio show that would feature the voices of men from inside San Quentin. His fifth try succeeded, to his surprise, when KFRC manager Bill Pabst acknowledged that it was an intriguing idea. During the Second World War, the radio show

"San Quentin on the Air" brought the voices of men serving time in San Quentin Prison to thousands of listeners outside the prison. On January 12, 1942, visitors came into San Quentin for the first broadcast, and the 5,000 men in custody felt like they were on trial before the public. The members of the band wore colourful uniforms donated by the San Rafael Sciots Lodge. The glee club members "begged, borrowed, or bleached" white shirts and duck pants. Hendricks's orchestra and a choir performed. Duffy provided short reflections between acts. The event caught the attention of Tin Pan Alley publishers, who sent eighteen to twenty-five songs per week to the radio show, hoping these songs would be included in the prison broadcast. "San Quentin on the Air" spread to more than 300 stations, and around 4,000 listeners' fan letters arrived in San Quentin weekly (Duffy and Jennings 1968, 234–43). This radio show provided a space for the public to listen to the incarcerated voices, besides promoting new songs by Tin Pan Alley songwriters.

Another California warden, Kenyon Judson Scudder (1890–1977) took a view similar to Duffy's. In 1952 he published a book titled *Prisoners Are People* that described his progressive penology. Scudder successfully argued against the completion of the partly built gun towers at the California Institution for Men at Chino, which opened in 1941. He also recommended that no inner fence be built around the buildings. In effect, this meant that the men in the prison could make their own decisions about whether to escape. George Briggs, a member of the prison board, explained that these changes at this minimum-security facility were motivated by its philosophy of freedom and autonomy:

The policy of the prison board is based on the concept that there can be no regeneration except in freedom. Rehabilitation must come from within the individual and not through coercion. With this principle in mind, the rehabilitative program of the prison system of California contemplates not only important education and vocational factors, but also, by and through classification and segregation, a gradual release from custodial restraint and a corresponding increase in personal responsibility and freedom of choice. (Scudder 1968, 28–29)

Scudder noted that the men in custody "have the same emotions and ambitions as other human beings. The mere fact that they have broken the law and are incarcerated while others go free does not stamp out those desires and ambitions" (5). This approach—building mutual respect between prison administrators and people in custody—contrasts sharply with punitive approaches toward imprisonment.

During his leadership at Chino, Scudder created a facility that recognized the dignity and potential worth of all imprisoned people. He initiated recreation activities for the men, including softball, ping pong, horseshoes, tennis, handball, volleyball, squash, and a favorite, croquet. An annual field day was held, and once, as a reward for good conduct, 200 Italian prisoners of war were bussed to Chino to participate. A Labor Day parade included twenty men from the livestock crew riding wild horses they had gentled,[18] fifteen floats that represented shops from the prison, including the vegetable garden crew, who exhibited their produce—cabbage, tomatoes, squash, onions, and "great bunches of luscious grapes set against a beautiful background of greenery" (225). The kitchen, cannery, and bakery combined to show fresh green salads, rolls, huge loaves of bread, and a sign from the cannery: "We Can Everything, But Our Boss Can't Can Us" (224–25). The Labor Day Parade was followed by a field meet, a football game, and the grand opening of a swimming pool.

On August 15, 1948, the pianist José Iturbi (1895–1980) gave an hour and forty-five-minute performance on a Baldwin concert grand piano in the Chino prison. Prior to the performance, 800 men completed a survey that asked them to choose their favourite selections from a long list. Iturbi "held them in the palm of his hand" (236), playing what they wanted to hear. After the performance, when Scudder asked the men if they should invite him back the following year, the men emphatically cried, "Yes! Yes!" Iturbi replied, "No, I will be back in six months" (235–36).

Over a period of ten years, Warden Scudder and his partner, Becky, hosted almost 1,000 incarcerated men in their home. With no guards attending, these normalizing interactions inside a home, with a crackling fire, singing, and a sense of freedom, brought the men new confidence, courage, and self-respect (232). Scudder's approach to creating agency, autonomy, and freedom within the constraints of prison, with music-making available for the men in custody, sharply differs from contemporary punitive administrative procedures. Additionally, at that point in history, someone sentenced to life was eligible for parole after seven and a half years; this is far different from the sentences of life without parole that are so common in this century.

In 1955, Missouri Governor Phil Donnelly (1891–1961) responded to a public desire for prison reform when he hired Colonel James Carter as the new director of prisons. Colonel Carter's approach was to include fair, firm, formal, and disciplined academic education, vocational training, and religious programming. When the Missouri Training Center for Men opened in Moberly in 1963, Chaplain Earl Grandstaff wanted to explore how a choir might affect rehabilitation. Prior to the opening of MTC, Chaplain Grandstaff had worked at a prison in Jefferson City, where he heard one of the incarcerated men, Leslie Sheard, harmonizing with a few other men. These singers were the start of the thirteen-member choir, all of whom were transferred to MTC. Support for this choir project came from Colonel Carter, the prison population, many people on the prison staff, and citizens from the local community. With the help of Leslie, Grandstaff auditioned men in the prison for vocal skill ability, but no formal musical training was required for membership. Through ear training and musical studies, they learned tone production, rhythms, vocal blend, and music appreciation with the goals of developing socialization, self-worth, communication, and discipline.

This forty-member choir, The Prodigals, rehearsed for ninety minutes five days a week and sang for Sunday services. They also rehearsed after evening meals, sometimes as late as 10 p.m., and they practised on weekends if needed (Richmiller 1992).

Grandstaff required a racially balanced group of singers. When a choir opening arose, they filled it so as to keep the racial balance, with singing ability a secondary priority. Some singers objected, and some staff members said the voices did not blend, but Chaplain Grandstaff gave an ultimatum—either singing with a racial balance or no singing in the chapel (18–19). The choir members overcame this issue and made things work. If a new member was initially unable to match pitch, he sang in the middle of some strong singers in his section. If he did not progress, he usually dropped out on his own (20).

A key part of the transformational power of this choir, as in the other music education programs in these twentieth-century prisons, was the social connections created between people inside and outside the institution. On Saturday evenings The Prodigals hosted church and community choirs for "Singspirations" inside the prison, where they performed for family and community members and joined in communal singing with everyone present. On November 27, 1963, 1,000 people attended the choir's first performance outside the prison: a community Thanksgiving service. The choir served as an incentive for good behaviour in the prison, and incarcerated men who travelled outside the prison were required to have a clean conduct record. The twenty-four choir members rotated through opportunities to travel to performances at colleges and churches, where they enjoyed a delicious meal as part of the outing. Eighteen to twenty choir members travelled out of prison at a time (81). They continued to address issues of racial segregation through these public performances by requiring that Black and white churches collaborate to host the choir, with the members of each congregation preparing food for the meal after the concert. Some churches withdrew their invitations due to this requirement.

Chaplain Grandstaff coached the men on how to interact appropriately at meals. After the performances, the singers sat with families in the community. Initially singers ate with families of their own skin colour, though the meals were eventually integrated. According to Grandstaff, some of the families in small towns were initially somewhat anxious, but by the end of the evening everyone was having a wonderful time and laughing, an accomplishment Grandstaff described as "another milestone," explaining, "We'd broken ground in a new place" (101).[19]

MTC also had a radio program called "Prisoners at Prayer," which began with The Prodigals singing their theme song, "No Man Is an Island." This radio program grew in popularity, and by March 21, 1964, it was being broadcast over seventeen stations throughout the Midwest. The Prodigals received many invitations to perform outside the prison. At these performances, the men in the choir demonstrated responsibility and showed they could be trusted. One of the venues they performed at was the J.W. "Blind" Boone Community Center in Columbia, Missouri, which sold alcohol. None of the choir members drank a drop of it (84). These opportunities provided a deep sense of normalization, improved the men's communication and social skills, and gave them an incentive to follow the prison rules. John, a former Prodigal choir member, reported:

> The choir kept us around real people and a real world when we would have been in the bastard world of a prison where inmates didn't stay realistic. Inmates do time in almost a semi-daze. They shut off what they don't want to think about. Basically, it's hard to draw them out. At all times, Chappie [Chaplain Grandstaff] and the choir kept us in the real world. I think that's important. They did not allow us to slip back into this prison game or semi-conscious state. And never allowed us the time to get bitter. I don't think I remember any choir member who ever left prison bitter. Instead of going out bitter, we came out trusting the world. (89)

Grandstaff's choir provides an example of how music-making, in this instance choral singing, kept the men in custody engaged and motivated to trust society, besides providing experiences that would support successful re-entry into post-prison life and building new social connections between Black and white people. As a result of these community connections, the prison received donations such as trees, shrubs, roses, perennials, a classical record collection, and greeting cards to encourage contact with family.

Twenty-nine years later, Mary Richmiller collected data from seventeen of the members, Chaplain Grandstaff, and selected prison staff through interviews and questionnaires. They reported that the choir had provided a sense of purpose, achievement, and recognition. Community involvement proved to be central to the men's increased self-esteem. The men in the prison reported feeling that they were valuable contributors to the community through their musical experiences and that participation in the choir increased their ability to focus on goals. They also credited the choir with helping them develop self-discipline as well as social and communication skills. With respect to how the choir prepared them for re-entry, one mentioned that it provided "freedom of spirit; a hopeful outlook; something to be proud of. Most of all, a sense of giving a pure gift of beauty" (Richmiller 1992, 35). Clearly, then, music-making can be a means for those who are incarcerated to provide others with beauty, in this case through choral singing. Richmiller's research indicates that when done right, group music-making can support re-entry, develop self-discipline, and humanize people once considered "the other."

In the first two-thirds of the twentieth century, many reports from across the US indicated support for music programs in prisons. Also, several administrators noted that musical communities were impactful for participants, for other people in the prison, and for public relations. These prison leaders supported musical communities and musical learning in their facilities. There is also some evidence that when prison administrators allowed music programs in their facilities, incarcerated people experienced personal growth, for those programs fostered hard work, self-discipline, self-reflection, emotional expression, creative communication, and positive self-identities, besides improving self-esteem. These programs promoted social growth for both incarcerated individuals and community members, leading to improved family relationships and a sense of being accepted by people outside the prison. Music-making also made society more aware of the humanity of people in custody. Such activities provided space for new friendships and improved teamwork skills. Visionary wardens have the power to support innovative music-making in their facilities, but without societal awareness of the harms that have occurred prior to and during incarceration, and without a reimagining of how to deal with the societal issues in which these harms are rooted, the evidence presented in this chapter will likely not bring about transformative change. Music-making can develop participants' self-esteem, sense of agency, and personal responsibility. Socially, music-making can create bridges between life inside and outside prison.

These points all relate to what the criminology literature calls desistance theory. Desistance refers to a person's cessation of criminal behaviour given a prior consistent pattern of offending. Many scholars suggest that desistance is multifaceted (Maruna 2001; McNeill 2006; Rocque 2017) and that it has three components: first, a period of non-offending; second, redefining oneself with a positive self-perception; and third, developing a sense of belonging to a community (McNeill 2014). Desistance needs to start while people are in custody and requires a transformation of societal attitudes, including forgiveness, reconciliation, and a sense of our common humanity. As described throughout this chapter, music-making is a tool for personal growth and for creating a new identity. For people in custody, such new identities can include musician, instrumentalist, guitarist, pianist, percussionist, singer, songwriter, choir member, or a host of other musical identities. Audience members, peers, and even family members may also perceive incarcerated individuals in these new ways. Such experiences of music-making are humanizing. A musical ensemble can create social connections between people in custody and people who are not, welcoming the former back into society (Cohen and Henley 2018). Music-making can motivate people to participate in other learning activities and help build social skills and social capital. Such growth can help create effective re-entry plans. The possibilities for growing collaborative communities of care through music-making in prisons, when rooted in mindful and appropriate pedagogy, are numerous.

Group music-making encourages incarcerated people to interact with one another, including with those they would not otherwise associate with. These interactions provide spaces for relationship-building within prison walls—an important aspect of reimagining identity as well as for effective re-entry. Even when incarcerated musicians are studying music or learning to play an instrument without direct interaction with others, the processes require agency and self-discipline as they explore musical genres of their choice. Additionally, songwriting and singing songs that epitomize one's life can serve as a means for narrative development, creating a deeper sense of self-identity (Cursley and Maruna 2015). These points are especially relevant, given that criminology researchers have largely accepted the idea that a transformation of one's self-narrative and the restoring of one's sense of agency are key elements of desistance and successful re-entry (Liem and Richardson 2014).

Although the examples of successful prison music programs in this chapter seem paltry given the huge carceral population in the US, they do suggest that music—both performing and creating it—provides unique opportunities for personal growth. Group singing helps people in custody feel connected to their personal emotions and build relationships with the broader society. As people we are "hardwired to connect," and music-making provides opportunities for both personal and social connections.

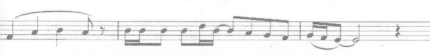

CHAPTER 3

"I ENCOURAGE EVERYONE TO STEP OUTSIDE THEIR COMFORT ZONE"

Developing Agency through Instrumental Music Education in Prisons

*It is important that music educators inside and outside of pris-*ons learn about their students' cultures. Building critical and sociopolitical awareness involves gaining an understanding of the challenges students face in a given environment. Incarcerated students' environments are restrictive by design, and that design involves the suppression, if not removal, of individual agency as well as the denial of social and cultural identity through the control of what they wear, how they can communicate with others, and how they can lead their lives. Fostering music-making skills can significantly mitigate the physical and psychological effects of this suppression of agency. Instrumental music-making entails learning techniques and coordinating psychomotor skills. It requires patience, self-discipline, and motivation. In effective instrumental programs in prisons, incarcerated students can easily notice their musical growth as they develop their performance skills. Those students also develop their ability to respond to instruction and create an identity as musical performers. These aspects of instrumental music-making help students grow personally; also, when performing with or for others, they promote social growth. In this chapter, through several case studies of instrumental music education programs in prisons, we highlight important elements of music education that develop a sense of autonomy and agency, sensitivity to others, and skills and habits of social responsiveness.

Music educator Jack Bowers worked at the Correctional Training Facility in Soledad, California, from 1980 to 2007.[1] In his instrumental music education programs, he established monthly band meetings in four different security locations in the prison. At these meetings the incarcerated musicians collaborated by creating rules to guide rehearsal and performance schedules, to manage the use of equipment and supplies, and to develop a shared understanding of what it means to be a part of a band. Bowers chaired these meetings. Each band had a designated leader, and there was a paid or volunteer person in custody who acted as the "band master," managing the band room operations under Bowers's guidance. Thus, the participants regulated, monitored, and managed the programs themselves. This system created a tradition of shared governance, eliminating most conflicts within the program.

The William James Association has contracted artists to work in California prisons, including Bowers, who has continued to work as a Senior Arts Mentor with that organization. Another noted artist with this organization was Henry Robinett, who taught guitar to men in custody in many different California prisons starting in 1993 (Carnes 2017, 7). In an interview with a journalist from *The Sun Magazine*, Robinett noted that caring does not exist in prison. He emphasized the vital need for society to care about people behind bars in order to improve harsh and broken prison systems. The racial tension in one of the prisons where he taught was so intense that a Black student dropped out of a band program because he was asked to share a trumpet with a white student. When white gang members found out about it, they told Robinett that "they can't have a white trumpet player putting his lips on an instrument that a black guy was playing" (Carnes 2017, 13). The Black gangs did not have a concern about the two men sharing a trumpet. However, if they had continued sharing a trumpet, "one of them could have gotten stabbed." So the Black student dropped out of the band program. Social dynamics are magnified in prisons, and stories like this one illustrate how tense relationships negatively impact learning and hinder growth.

One of the longest-term paid instrumental music educators in a US prison was Charles Musgrave, who taught in the Indiana State Prison (ISP) in Michigan City for twenty-two years, from 1974 to 1995.[2] Important to his long tenure was his ability to connect what was going on inside the prison musically with the outside world. For example, his musicians had a performance broadcast on a local South Bend radio show. Charles Bickel (1910–2008), the president of Conn-Selmer, Inc., a maker of band instruments, heard that performance. He donated forty instruments to the prison concert band, an indication of the importance he attached to offering instrumental band instruction to adults who had not played an instrument before. Thus supplied with instruments, Musgrave was able to offer music ensembles in additional styles, including soul, rock, and country, as well as a men's choir. Building on these connections with people outside the prison, he invited political leaders to attend performances in the prison. On seeing and hearing Musgrave's musicians, they made recommendations that additional music programs be started in other Indiana prisons. One politician, State Representative Mary Kay Budak, clearly impressed by what she heard, compared Musgrave's four-voice vocal group accompanied by a five-piece ensemble, "Spectrum," to the Temptations (Stattman 1982).

Part of Musgrave's new pedagogical approach involved a creative reward system in conjunction with musical performances. This innovation had the full support of Warden Jack Duckworth, without which it is unlikely that such a system would have been implementable, sustainable, or effective. Over two or three weeks, a number of instrumental groups performed in a series of seven concerts, including a concert band, a jazz band, a rock band, and a country band. The reward system allowed men who had no disciplinary reports to attend the concert and bring one outside guest to the performance. This alone would likely have been a strong motivator. However, the warden allowed an additional motivating factor: the men in custody would be able to sit right next to their guest, and many of them held hands with their loved ones during the performance. This was a striking exception to what we have seen across prisons, given that interactions between an incarcerated individual and a visitor usually take place with physical separation enforced by a booth and a window. Each guest was screened on their way into the prison, and the auditorium held about 300 people. Musicians who performed could also have their guest attend the night performance if it was their cell house's turn to come to the concert. While it is unlikely that it was the only factor, it is compelling that during the fourteen years that the concerts were offered, there were no prison riots. This creative reward system offered by the music education program cultivated a sense of agency, confidence, and pride, besides supporting responsible and pro-social behaviour.

The relationship that develops between an instrumental leader and their incarcerated student can facilitate personal and musical growth. One musician in Musgrave's program, Red McHenry, chose the trombone because he was told it would take more work to learn to play that instrument compared to other options. After about two years of study, Musgrave encouraged him to play a solo at one of the performances.

Although nervous, Red gave the performance his best effort. After the performance, Red shared with Musgrave that the reason he robbed banks was not for the money, but rather for the thrill he felt while doing it. After he successfully performed the solo, he came off stage and told Musgrave he would never rob a bank again. He said that the high he experienced from performing the solo was the biggest he had ever enjoyed, better than robbing banks and better than doing drugs (Charles Musgrave, email to Mary Cohen, January 7, 2021). These sorts of transformative experiences are possible when incarcerated students are given opportunities to develop autonomy and self-esteem through the pedagogical act of learning an instrument, exploring various musical literatures, and sharing that journey with others through the act of performance.

The program attracted attention from musicians. For example, noted jazz educator and saxophonist Jamey Aebersold visited the Indiana State Prison and donated his jazz play-along records to Musgrave for his students to use.[3] Yet however successful music programs can be in improving behaviour and concentration, and instilling a positive identity, external factors can rapidly end or drastically change programs. When prison administrators shifted away from a rehabilitative approach and members of the general public became less open to educational avenues, the state was less supportive of the music program, arguing that it was not punitive enough and that funds were lacking to hire a replacement for Musgrave after he left the job (Charles Musgrave, personal communication to author Mary Cohen, November 11, 2019).

Bowers, Robinett, and Musgrave all received support during the height of their programming. Institutional support, as illustrated in these case studies, is vital if there is to be effective music programming in prisons. These three musical leaders all had to deal with challenges within the facility such as prison rules and social tensions. Navigating these challenges is part of the toolset for musicians working in prisons; fostering good relations with the warden and staff is vital to help navigate both prison leadership and political changes.

As Musgrave once told a reporter: "I encourage everyone to step outside their comfort zone. That's the only way you'll accomplish something" ("Prisoners Keep Time" 1984, 5). All leaders of musical experiences make pedagogical choices that have the potential to support new growth, empower learners' identities, and create meaningful social connections. Given the diversity of musical styles in the US, and the wide range of learners' interests and needs, music educators can be most effective if they have a clear idea about why they are teaching in any context, a clear understanding of their own social and musical identities as they relate to their purpose, clear intentions for teaching a particular style or composition, learning activities to develop students' awareness of their personal and musical identities, and affirming ways to challenge their students. Effective music educators encourage their students to try new things and learn often difficult skills; they also develop meaningful relationships with their learners that inform their planning, instruction, and assessment.

Researchers from the fields of education and music education have developed teaching frameworks that develop learner agency, supporting individual students and group learning. Culturally relevant pedagogy (CRP), created by US pedagogical theorist and teacher educator Gloria Ladson-Billings, is perhaps the most relevant to music-making in prisons. After realizing that many studies regularly associated African American students with a "deficit model" of learning with terms such as disadvantaged, at-risk, and underachieving, she argued that there was a lack of language that connected academic excellence with African American students. She set out to discover what was effective with African American learners and what happened in classrooms where teachers were successful with their pedagogies. She defines culturally relevant pedagogy as:

> a pedagogy of opposition not unlike critical pedagogy but specifically committed to collective, not merely individual, empowerment. Culturally relevant pedagogy rests on three criteria or

propositions: (a) students must experience academic success; (b) students must develop and/or maintain cultural competence; and (c) students must develop a critical consciousness through which they challenge the status quo of the current social order. (1995, 160)

By cultural competence, Ladson-Billings (2014) was referring to "the ability to help students appreciate and celebrate their cultures of origin" (75) while learning about at least one additional culture. Such competence allows learners to develop deeper agency with respect to their own ethnic identity. In a music classroom, teachers who develop an understanding of their students' cultural backgrounds can make effective pedagogical choices with respect to musical styles and artists. With respect to challenging the current social status quo, such efforts are impossible if teachers and students are unaware of the complexities and truth of the history of colonialization, slavery, and targeted criminalization in the US. Two scholars who study race, Django Paris and H. Samy Alim, have developed the CRP framework into what they call culturally sustaining pedagogy (CSP).[4]

Because the number of people of colour in the carceral system is extremely disproportionate to their presence in society, culturally sustaining pedagogies are important for music educators to employ, particularly music educators who teach in prisons. Paris and Alim note that they have experienced first-hand the racially discriminatory contexts of schooling in the US throughout their lives, first as students, then as teachers (2017, 4). They argue that the purpose of school has long been to assimilate white colonial settlers at the expense, and harm, of people of colour. These experiences and their research inform their efforts to decentre whiteness in the school curriculum. They suggest that the purpose of schooling in pluralist societies is to foster and sustain literate, linguistic, and cultural pluralism toward positive social transformation. Teachers who adopt CSP practices emphasize affirming interactions with their students and establish an anti-racist pedagogy that actively pushes back against notions of white supremacy (1). CSP is a fairly new pedagogical approach in music education, and a strong need exists for pre-service and in-service music educators to learn about and implement CSP in schools and in prisons.

Ladson-Billings (2017, 143) responded to Paris and Alim's development of CRP by noting that cultural competence is "the 'misunderstood' aspect of CRP." Her understanding of the term "culture" is rooted in her studies in anthropology. She describes culture as "an amalgamation of human activity, production, thought, and belief systems" (Ladson-Billings 2014, 75) and includes all components of human endeavours—feelings, attitudes, thoughts, and perceptions. Culture, in their view, is fluid and dynamic and includes ethics, ways of being, world views, and nuances that take deliberate study to learn. A culturally competent teacher values all cultures and understands that all students have culture. It follows that cultural competency is a vital starting point for teaching and learning. Ladson-Billings (2017, 145–46) noted that developing students' critical consciousness has been the most neglected element of CRP.

Neuroscience research teaches us that cognitive, emotional, and social-psychological abilities mature at different ages and that psychosocial maturity or one's ability to practise self-restraint in emotional situations is not fully developed until youth are in their mid- to late twenties (Icenogle et al. 2019). One of the most harmful effects of punitive approaches to crime occurs through the incarceration of youth. Developmental science findings suggest that eighteen- to twenty-five-year-olds are similar to teenagers in their psychological abilities and brain maturation. Variations in developmental changes between early and late adolescence, and from late adolescence to young adulthood, require us to provide special care, protections, and opportunities for healthy development. Researchers suggest that young adulthood should be its own developmental stage in the justice system (Casey et al. 2020). Yet youth and young adults in the US have repeatedly been locked up, sometimes placed with adult populations, sometimes with sentences that last decades or longer, and sometimes in solitary confinement. Pedagogical approaches such as CSP provide teachers inside and outside prisons with a means to contribute to positive learning experiences for all youth and young adults, particularly students of colour.

For eight years, Megan Holkup taught junior high, high school, GED students, and graduate students in both graphic communications and music at the Marmot High School in the Youth Correctional Center in Mandan, North Dakota, where the teachers worked to fold life skills and social skills into treatment, personal interactions, and education. Her maximum class size was eight students, with a rolling enrolment. Holkup's teaching philosophy incorporated culturally relevant and sustaining pedagogies; this entailed co-creating individual goals that aligned with the schedule for their time in custody and that emphasized their successes and learning styles.

One of Holkup's aims was to teach her students to be independent learners so that they would be able to teach themselves when they left the school. She emphasized trust in the musical process and relationship-building. She taught piano skills, rhythm skills, reading and writing notation, music theory applied to their goals, audio mixing and editing, and arranging. In each class, she and her students worked on one of these musical elements as a group. Students then focused on their own individual goals, such as playing three songs on the guitar or composing a piece. All her students met their first goal and then worked to complete additional goals. They also identified long-term music-specific goals in their lives. An example of one of her students' long-term goals was "I will write songs for guitar/vocals and record an LP."

In conversations with students about establishing their goals, Holkup noticed that they often used the phrase "I want to," but when she repeated their ideas back to them, she used the words "I will," encouraging them to be more self-confident that they could achieve the goal they had set for themselves. They discussed the difference between "I want" and "I will," and she encouraged them to establish measurable goals.

In an effort to connect with her students' personal environment, Holkup asked her students to complete a survey each day to reflect on their levels of distress and what, if anything, helped them deal with the pressures they felt. They reported that writing lyrics and arranging and recording original music were some of the most important activities that helped them work through their stresses and supported their personal growth. The students wanted to put themselves into their creations to make them more original.

When reflecting on the differences between teaching students in the public schools in North Dakota and teaching system-impacted youth at Marmot, Holkup remarked that her students at Marmot may not have had the same success in traditional school music education programs as they did in her classes. Students who have dealt with major setbacks and low self-esteem felt like failures when they were told they played wrong notes. This emphasis on making mistakes can lead to roadblocks. The youth at Marmot had not yet built the resilience to view mistakes as practice hurdles. Holkup's efforts were rooted in meeting the students where they were, supporting their strengths, and inviting them to connect to the musical content on a personal level (Megan Holkup, email message to Mary Cohen, November 21, 2018). In Holkup's classes, the students learned to practise, used critical thinking skills to figure out what and how to improve, focused on the areas that challenged them, and pursued tasks until they had gained proficiency.

Holkup taught her students how to teach themselves using ideas based on culturally sustaining frameworks. From the first day of class, she worked to connect with them individually and build trusting relationships, affirming their strengths and encouraging them to become independent learners.

Holkup decided she would have a greater opportunity to make systemic change by working as a training director instead of a music instructor at Marmot. In this new role, she facilitates her employees' professional development and instructs her staff that their specialty does not need to be confined to their title. For example, a new Marmot employee saw a guitar next to her desk and inquired about playing music with the youth, not realizing that Holkup had once been the music teacher at the school. Another staff member expressed an interest in learning to play the drums. Holkup supported these employees' interests in connecting with the youth through music-making and modelling lifelong learning. Just as she encouraged her students to be lifelong learners, she supports her staff to have that same mentality and to use their imaginations to bring their gifts into their work and to model how music-making is a lifelong learning process (Megan Holkup, phone call to Mary Cohen, January 12, 2021).

A second example of instrumental music education for youth in custody demonstrates the success of strength-based and culturally sustaining pedagogies. The Gardner Betts Juvenile Center in Austin, Texas, offers a comprehensive youth program, including a high school credit-bearing guitar class. Most youth complete the required treatment, and as a result they are released from custody and do not go into the adult state prison system. Many of the students in the guitar class have come in with no previous guitar skills and have learned to play guitar successfully. As soon as the instructors notice their students overcoming technical or musical obstacles, they affirm them (Marcum 2014).

Jeremy Osborne is a guitar instructor at the centre. He worked to build a positive relationship with his student David Fredrick. David could already play guitar when he was placed in Gardner. Initially, he was not open to Osborne's instructions, but eventually the two built a positive rapport and David learned to play collegiate-level repertoire. However, he was not keeping up with the facility's treatment requirements, and the staff told him he could not play guitar in the facility until he participated in his requirements for treatment. Without following the staff's ultimatum, he could have been transferred to a different youth centre that lacked the wealth of programming that Gardner Betts offered. Osborne affirmed David's remarkable musical skills and encouraged him to make the necessary steps to improve himself. He did not know whether he would see David in the upcoming fall term. Over the summer, David did complete the required treatment, and while waiting for Osborne to return in the fall, he created a full-size paper guitar with strings, frets, a sound hole, a rosette decoration, and a display stand using the only materials available to him: copy paper, yarn, and tape (Hinsley, Marcum, and Osborne 2016, 36). Through asset-based and relationship-building instruction, David was motivated to work hard to repair what had traumatized him in order to build his self-efficacy and support his own betterment.

The guitar program's guiding principle is expressive performance. Through a nine-level comprehensive curriculum created in consultation with music education professor Robert Duke at the University of Texas at Austin, the instructors facilitate group learning that scaffolds beginners successfully, accommodating their skill development. Initial compositions include two-note melodies played expressively; instructors then use midi files to add beats while students play artfully with good tone. They collect lists of songs the students enjoy and develop their ability to play by ear as they build literacy skills. The instructors work to create supportive spaces for their students to build identities, create something special, and feel pride in their accomplishment (Hinsley, Marcum, and Osborne 2016, 37). Osborne says that he never quite knows how students will respond during instruction, so he approaches learning processes with flexibility and relationship-building. Ninety percent of the guitar students indicated they had no previous associations with any learning success prior to their experiences in this program.

In these examples, positive reinforcement of musical learning led to behavioural adjustments for men and youth in custody. Women in custody have their own learning needs. Over the past three and a half decades the number of incarcerated women in the US has increased over 700 percent, outpacing the increase in men during the same period by 50 percent. This increase is rooted in policy changes that have led to more intense sentencing (Datchi and Ancis 2017, 2). Because sentences are getting longer, more women are now in custody.[5] This extreme rise also affects children and families, as many women are the primary caregivers for their children. Parental incarceration creates chaos in children's lives, including negative emotional and behavioural consequences and economic hardship (Seymour and Hairston 2001). Around 60 percent of incarcerated women have two children (Glaze and Maruschak 2008).

An institution outside Anchorage, Alaska, is attempting to address the rise in women's incarceration rates with an approach that includes music education. The administrators' philosophy at Hiland Mountain Correctional Center, a facility in Eagle River, Alaska, is that incarceration is meant to be a growth opportunity, not punishment. The Hiland Mountain Women's String Orchestra meets this goal explicitly. Learning to play a string instrument requires self-discipline, consistent practice, patience to develop fine motor skills, and precision in order to play in a group. This women's orchestra started in 2003 when Pati Crofut was seeking membership in a beginning adult orchestra and Janice Weiss, the education director at Hiland, was looking for educational programming for the women's prison. Together they formed a not-for-profit organization, Arts on the Edge. Alaskans who read in the *Anchorage Daily News* about the new orchestra donated instruments and some funds to help start the program. The initial group consisted of eight beginning string players. These women met on Saturdays and practised on their own during the week. The women in the orchestra gave their first performance on June 12, 2004. They initially had two concerts per year, but decided it was too difficult to learn enough literature for two annual concerts. Because their performances include a charity fundraiser, they chose to have their annual concert in December, when the community is more generous in providing donations.

The former superintendent at Hiland, Dean Marshall, described how the orchestra is one of the more transformative activities available inside this prison, in part because it has allowed the women to make social and musical connections with the arts community, including Grammy Award–winning American cellist Zuill Bailey, who performed as a soloist with the orchestra in 2012. Concert audiences have been so large that the orchestra has offered two separate outside concerts for three hundred people each, plus a concert for incarcerated women. Such large audiences provide opportunities for more of the Anchorage community to come into the prison and hear the women perform. Bailey was so impressed with the experience that he continues to perform solo concerts in the prison each September, often bringing musicians from the Sitka Summer Music Festival.

When the women are practising, Marshall notes, they are not getting in trouble. The women learn that they have a large responsibility to themselves and to others in the group. A former violist in the orchestra, Sally Elizabeth Woodson, explained that the orchestra changed the atmosphere inside the prison. The practices and performances contrast sharply with the daily mundane tasks the women are required to do, indicating that not all experiences inside the prison are growth opportunities. Their music education provides more autonomy and an outlet for self-expression. She notes that it is liberating, inspirational, and spiritual.[6]

Many family members eagerly attend the annual December public concerts; so do formerly incarcerated orchestra members and other supporters from the community. These performances blend community and professional musicians with the women's orchestra—sometimes as many as forty performers in two or three orchestras. Financial support comes from the community through ticket sales to this annual performance and sales of crafts made by the incarcerated women.[7] Co-performers and audience members make in-person connections with the women inside the Hiland facility. These connections have varied outcomes—negative, neutral, or positive—depending on a host of issues. For example, some people in custody who do not have outside visitors at the concert may feel lonely or sad. As music educators, the more we understand our students' perspectives and feelings, the more responsive we can be to their needs. This is particularly important inside prisons when some students have guests attend performances and others do not. Our ability to be sensitive to students' inner lives influences the learners' self-efficacy and the possibilities of new and renewed social connections.

Kathryn Hoffer, orchestra teacher at Hiland from 2015 to 2020, used to play for the December Hiland performances prior to taking the role as teacher. She was touched each time she played for these events. In 2015, Hoffer signed a contract with the Alaska Department of Corrections for her position as orchestra leader. Such state funding is currently atypical for music education in US prisons, yet institutional and government support is necessary for successful music programs.[8] The State of Alaska pays Hoffer's salary through its education budget, but this program still needs private funds for many other expenses such as bringing in guest artists and purchasing and maintaining instruments. Some outside musicians make generous contributions to the organization. For example, Nancy Strelau, the orchestra conductor at Nazareth College in Rochester, New York, willingly offered to compose "The Journey" for the December 2018 performance. Strelau and two students paid for their own travel to Anchorage to attend rehearsals in August 2018.[9]

With respect to teaching experiences, Hoffer noted that the class itself is like any other orchestra situation, and her leadership of the prison orchestra is similar to how she taught in the schools. However, the women have jobs, court visits, treatment programs, and other issues that occasionally contribute to poor attendance. Hoffer found pieces to challenge the players who are ready and who want more difficult literature.

I (Mary Cohen) attended two orchestra concerts on December 2, 2017, inside the Hiland Correctional Facility. At the rehearsal on Friday, the day before the concert, many players, guests and incarcerated women wore long-sleeved green T-shirts labelled "Arts on the Edge." On the day of the concert, all performers wore concert black clothes, all of which were donated. In the fall they have a dress selection night where their classroom is converted into a dress shop with two dressing rooms. The women put together their outfits for the concert. Arts on the Edge purchases tights, stockings, and what they need to complete their "look." Once all the clothes are labelled, the executive director of Arts on the Edge, Pati Crofut, takes the dresses to a dry cleaner that donates its services. The assembled outfits are brought to Hiland one or two days ahead of the concert and are collected immediately after the concert. It is a rare experience for someone incarcerated to change out of their prison uniform into formal attire. This musical community in prison may be the only one that allows musicians in custody and outside volunteer musicians to dress alike for a performance, symbolizing their common humanity and united musical voice.

The beginning and advanced orchestras performed the first concert for an incarcerated audience of thirty-five men who were in a Transformational Learning Community at Hiland and about 100 incarcerated women. The prison staff keep the women and men separate within this facility, as they did in the concert audience. In this instance, musical performance provided a bridge between men and women in custody and a reason to stretch the rules, for it was too difficult for the orchestra to perform three separate concerts for women, men, and outside guests. Seven correctional officers stood around the edges of the gym, along with Superintendent Gloria Johnson, Pati Crofut, and four outside guests. This first concert lasted about an hour. A man in custody wept during the first piece, "Melody" by Antonín Dvořák.

Armen Ksajikian, the principal cellist of the Los Angeles Chamber Orchestra, is a frequent guest of the Sitka Summer Arts Festival. He has played in 2,000 films, including movies directed by Steven Spielberg. The Hiland women appreciate him and asked him to be the soloist. Five women spoke between selections. Hoffer asked them to reflect on what inspired them about music. One shared her reflection at the concert:

> To get a deeper sense of the question "how does music inspire you?" I looked up "inspire" and it means "to exert an animating, enlivening, or exalting influence upon." Exalting is a great word; a raising up in dignity. We use sporks at meal service here. A spork is neither an effective fork nor an effective spoon, so many of us resort to eating with our hands for efficiency (I do this). This is just one example of the degradation in an environment such as Hiland that erodes modesty and couth. Music, in this classical sense especially, can elevate this bleak, degrading trudge up into the airy atmosphere, not in some elitist, out-of-reach way, but in an omnipresent way like the flowers planted all around the institution in the summer. Beauty and class refine and restore our sophistication a little bit. They exalt. Playing in the orchestra allows me to tap into exaltation, rising up to a better view, where I see that I am capable of much more than I realize. (Hiland Orchestra performer)

This incarcerated musician's reflection indicates that the music education experience was a tool to remedy the degrading experiences she had encountered in the prison environment. The musical rehearsals and performances allowed her to rise above the humiliation and disgrace of prison life and inspired her toward a more authentic self-realization. The last orchestra member who spoke to the incarcerated audience said: "Hope you enjoy your stay at Hiland!" That gave the audience a good laugh.

The second performance was for an outside audience of about 250 people. When the orchestra program began in 2003, the prison administrators rented chairs for the audience members. Eventually, Arts on the Edge purchased chairs and donated them to the prison, so they have adequate seating for the audience members.

The six-member beginners' orchestra performed first and included one woman who had been released one week prior.[10] In most prison contexts, it would be quite rare for prison administrators to grant special permission for someone to return to prison who had just been released. It is also rare for someone to *want* to come back inside prison immediately after release. This player's dedication and the support of the prison administration are both evidence of this program's deep value. For audience members from the general public, seeing a formerly incarcerated orchestra member come back into the prison to play a concert increases their awareness of the profound social value of this music education experience.

Armen Ksajikian performed four solo pieces accompanied by pianist Susan Wingrove Reed. Ksajikian played with both orchestras and was featured with the advanced orchestra on Brian Balmages's "It Takes One to Tango." Eight string players and a percussionist from the Anchorage Symphony Orchestra joined the advanced ensemble. The beginning and advanced orchestras played two different sets, and the orchestras performed together at the end. The concert ended with a double surprise: an encore performance of Henry Mancini's "Pink Panther Theme," during which a person dressed up like the Pink Panther danced through the aisles, giving the audience members great laughter and joy. The members described how they felt the support of the audience, pride in a job well done, and sadness at ending what had been a huge project. Arts on the Edge provided $100 stipends to each outside player, and according to Pati Crofut, many of these musicians returned their cheques to Crofut, for they found the project valuable and wished to donate their time. There is an adult amateur intermediate-level string orchestra in the community. Several released orchestra members have tried to participate in it; however, their jobs and family activities have tended to prevent their full participation.

With respect to recruiting and retention, Superintendent Gloria Johnson chooses the new beginning orchestra members after women who are interested in joining complete a form. Johnson checks that the women will be incarcerated through the December concert and that they have had no disciplinary reports in the previous six months. She ascertains whether any women have a musical background and shares that information with Hoffer.

Retention is another challenge. It is difficult to play a string instrument. The new players need self-discipline, perseverance, and a positive attitude. One year forty applied, thirty were approved to join the beginning orchestra, and twenty-five performed in a concert. Another year eighteen were in the class and fifteen in the concert. In 2017 the beginning orchestra started with sixteen and ended with six.

Changes in sentencing laws impact orchestra membership. When Alaska Senate Bill 91 removed incarceration for petty crimes, the prison population diminished; however, more petty crimes occurred. Senate Bill 54 reversed 91, so it is anticipated that more people will be going into prison. Sometimes women who are on a federal sentence are transferred to another state. Clearly, a wide range of issues affect membership in a prison-based musical ensemble.

Although full-time music educators inside US prisons were more common prior to the rise of mass incarceration, music educators are occasionally contracted through a state's Department of Corrections to come into a facility and create a program, like Hoffer did in Alaska. In other countries with lower rates of both incarceration and recidivism, full-time music educators are employed in prisons. For example, in 2019 in Norway, a country with an incarceration rate of 49 people per 100,000 compared to the US's 639 people per 100,000, forty-two prisons provided music programs funded by the government.

The very fact that a music leader is external to a prison system may better enable change within a system as well as in society. As these individuals discuss the criminal legal system with people in their communities, more people learn about problems within prison systems. The power dynamics within prisons—among people in custody as well as between incarcerated individuals and staff—may create difficulties when an incarcerated person takes charge of music programming. One woman who played in the Hiland orchestra mentioned that she tried directing the other women in a prison choir and it was "nightmare-ish" to lead; her experience telling other incarcerated women what to do did not go over well.

In this chapter we have examined case studies that illustrate how music-making in prisons instills a sense of agency and autonomy in the learners, thus creating a deeper responsiveness. It is no wonder that people in custody within punitive systems, where the primary emphasis is on security, end up struggling with re-entry into the community. When people in custody encounter opportunities to build their agency in productive and meaningful ways, they can more effectively build the self-efficacy they require to live a fulfilling life. Learning to play a musical instrument is an effective way to grow personally, develop agency, and create social responsiveness, whether playing with or for others.

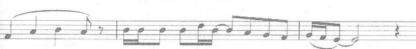

CHAPTER 4

"THEIR SINGING SAVED ME"
Social Awareness through Choral Singing

*C*horal singing is a learned skill requiring no external tools, which removes some of the barriers associated with instrumental music-making. In terms of logistics, vocal programs in prisons are easier to initiate and sustain than instrumental programs because group singing usually does not require instruments; this eases security concerns when outside instructors are entering and exiting prisons and removes issues of instrument storage inside prisons.

Choral singing provides space for a broader social awareness of the humanity of people in prison in two ways: through embodied experiences and sung words. In this chapter we offer contemporary examples of choral singing in prisons that support our contention that music-making provides opportunities for personal and social growth, as well as social awareness of the problems of prisons.

Singing engages the human body in ways that are different from playing an instrument. When singing together in a choir, people create choral sound; they *are* the musical agents. Using just their own bodies, choir members learn to attune with one another's voices, paying attention to the syllabic rhythmic breakdown, matching vowels, and working toward tonal balance and vocal blend.

Group singing or the "somatic factor" happens at individual and communal levels (Cohen 2007a, 20–22, 224–65). The human body is each singer's instrument and requires breath management, bodily alignment, and vocal phonation. Variables include participants' attitudes, physical health, feelings, intentions, and aspirations, as well as contextual and environmental factors; all of these play a role in each person's individual experience of music-making in a choir. Personal embodiment includes individual experiences of the muscular, circulatory, nervous, and respiratory systems, as well as thoughts and emotions.

Choral singing helps develop a sense of community and social embodiment; often this is magnified through sung texts as the participating choral singers and listeners develop a shared understanding through musical experiences and through singing and listening to different languages. Social embodiment includes awareness of these ideas expressed through text as well as interactions with other people. When people sing together, they listen, attune, connect, sing in unison and harmony with others, and perform for others. Choir participants create a communal body through rehearsals and performances. Together, choir members work toward mutual responsiveness, both with others in the group and for those who are listening. When we sing, we can express our humanity in creative ways that involve melodies, harmonies, rhythms, forms, and text. With effective leadership, group members learn to be respectful and nurturing of the social connections that happen non-verbally and verbally throughout their time together.

As people sing together, the sound produced lies along a continuum between unified blend and disjointed voices. If a unified blend is desired, the individuals in a choir practise singing in such a way that their individual voices match the pitch, quality, and volume of the other voices. Choir members learn to become sensitive to the relationships among the sounds of their voices in the acoustic environment. Vocal acousticians refer to aspects of this phenomenon as the "self-to-other ratio" (Ternström 1999, 3563–74). A deeper awareness of how one's voice blends with a group may also serve as a reference point for people as they practise welcoming others into their communities. Choral singing allows individuals to interact directly with others without an instrument as an intermediary and can be a step toward learning to cooperate with others. For people with narcissistic personalities, this lesson runs contrary to their perception of themselves as more important than the people around them. An Oakdale inside singer reported, "My second concert with the choir was a way for me to not be so self-centred" (OCC 2011). Choral singing in prisons allows opportunities for cooperation, self-expression, and deeper insight into others' experiences.

Another aspect of the somatic factor of singing is the influence of singing on well-being. Research studies indicate that choral singing provides psychophysical, social, and emotional benefits (Clements-Cortés 2015, 7–12). Specifically, singing reduces stress, strengthens the immune system, aids in relaxation, and improves breathing. Group singing improves mood, increases positive feelings, increases happiness, increases energy, decreases pain, improves self-esteem, develops a sense of collective belonging, builds friendships, and decreases loneliness. These positive outcomes of group singing can be especially beneficial for people in custody.

Compared to the general population, people in prison often have greater health needs (Sturup-Toft et al. 2018, 15–23). Incarcerated individuals suffer from a variety of health issues, including mental health challenges, drug and alcohol addiction, nutrition deficiencies, and negative outcomes from trauma. Fundamental to public health is the reduction of health inequalities. The state carries the responsibility for the well-being and health of people who are in custody. Yet Dr. Christine

Montross, Professor of Psychiatry and Human Behavior at Brown University and a practising in-patient psychiatrist, argues that incarceration in the US make people sicker with respect to both their physical and mental health (Montross 2020). Choral singing can directly improve the health of people in custody, but this is limited by the harmful outcomes of incarceration.

Breathing, phonating, singing texts, and attuning oneself to others all reawaken a sense of our physicality on both individual and communal levels. In prisons, where people are separated from society, the embodied experiences of singing together with people from outside the prison and performing for guests who attend concerts create spaces for transformation for both people in custody and people from the community.

In most choral songs, people vocalize words (Cohen 2007a, 18–20). The choral singing experience thus involves listening to words and experiencing an interplay of rhythm, melody, harmony, form, and expressive qualities through verbal language. These communal expressions of words and music can create opportunities for individual growth, depending on each choir member's motivation for learning. For the group, communal meanings derive from the shared experience of singing the messages of the songs they are learning.

The verbal aspect of choral singing can build literacy skills by providing opportunities for participants to learn and practise vocabulary in their native tongue, to explore world languages, and to experience a variety of lyrical forms and ideas in songs. Such cognitive growth can strengthen mental well-being and provide new avenues of inquiry and expression. Sung words may provide opportunities for personal reflection, and song lyrics can inspire ideas for original songs. Designing performances as musical developments of verbal themes—for example, "Peace and Place," "Light in the Darkness," "Finding Hope," "Remember: Be Love,"—can prompt reflection and discussion among singers and audience members.[1] The addition of words to musical expression can be a powerful stimulant for emotional expression.

For instance, the Oakdale Community Choir, in its first concert season, performed a song called "Homeward Bound." Prior to the start of the choir, I (Mary Cohen) held an introductory meeting with men in the prison to introduce the project. I brought a copy of the score to "Homeward Bound" to show them an example of a song and to ascertain how they would feel about singing lyrics that express a longing to return to their home and a desire to be unbound. I did not know how long each incarcerated individual's sentence was, and I wondered whether their separation from home and family might make the song too painful. They agreed this song would be appropriate for the choir, and after learning to sing it, one member wrote that he could not get the song out of his head: "Every time we sing this song, I feel the desire to cry" (OCC 2009). For this man, singing these lyrics about the longing for home was emotionally powerful. In a male prison, confessing that you feel like crying might be considered a risky and brave thing to do.[2] This example signifies the subtle yet impactful role of singing: how lyrics set to a beautiful melody can unlock feelings that men in prison may repress, and how a choir inside the prison provides a place to be brave enough to express those feelings.

Fall and winter holidays are especially difficult for people in custody. One incarcerated choir member, Tom Sheldon, shared the following reflection on the holiday song, "Celebrate Me Home," performed at the Oakdale December 2009 concert:

> "Celebrate Me Home" means more to me now than ever. In my mind it's a plea to God to reunite me with my family, as if the act of celebration can transport me back home. It's a sad, yearning, but also hopeful song. The closer we get to the holidays, the greater the sense of loss and separation for me. Part of that is from knowing my wife is alone and lonely through the holidays. We both know we'll survive the separation another year, but each year seems harder than the last. That's most likely an illusion of proximity; last year's aches have subsided. Still, we're aging, and

it seems to me that my wife is struggling harder than ever. I want
so much to comfort her. So, please, celebrate me home.

The song gave Tom pause to consider how difficult it is for him
to be apart from his wife over the Christmas holiday. He reflected on
the marital separation he had experienced, which he felt more deeply
during the Christmas season. As he read these words aloud to the incarcerated and community audiences, those listening had the opportunity
to feel a connection to the difficulties he and his wife had experienced
by living apart due to incarceration.[3]

Seeds for social change through choral singing are rooted in both
somatic and word factors. Embodied vocal expressions through choral
singing can take on deep meaning both for individuals in prisons and for
people outside of prisons. People in prison live apart from their home
communities in a situation where they have little or no autonomy; many
face exceedingly long sentences, including life without parole. Musical
communities within prisons provide some measure of agency; they
also build a bridge between societies outside and inside prison walls.
People outside of prisons can develop social awareness of prison issues
by listening to certain sung lyrics. The metaphors within songs can be
a medium for expressing incarcerated singers' personal feelings and
experiences. Words sung can illustrate the life experiences of people in
custody and their families, providing a space for deeper social awareness of the everyday challenges incarcerated individuals face.

Music leaders in prisons can increase social awareness in small and
large ways, but they may also unknowingly contribute to inequitable
and oppressive social structures that are at the root of the prison industrial complex. It is important for artistic leaders in prisons to grasp the
delicate balance between providing meaningful experiences and repli-
cating, perpetuating, or complying with broken systems.

One choral leader who has spent her life working toward meaningful
social change through singing, applying instructional practices similar

to culturally sustaining pedagogy, is Catherine Roma. Roma has developed choral programs in Ohio prisons for more than three decades, and her work continued alongside the rise of mass incarceration. When she received support from prison administrators, she has broadened social awareness of the humanity and artistry of men and women in custody.[4]

While working as a full-time assistant professor at Wilmington in 1993, Dean Batiuk asked Roma to start two choirs within prisons. For two years, Roma led "New Souls A-Risin'" in London Correctional Institution (LCI) in Ohio. LCI presented a variety of challenges related to space, scheduling, and lack of attention to the learning needs of the men in the prison. The prison had no green spaces, and the outdoor recreation space was a large outdoor cement cage. There were limited rooms available for group programming; the three full-time chaplains struggled to find spaces for their own offerings, which made it all the more difficult for Roma to find a room for the New Souls A-Risin' Choir to meet and practise. Administrative requests went unfulfilled, and responses to her requests were often harsh. For example, when the African American students in LCI wrote a letter to Dean Batiuk asking for more African American content and Black teachers to instruct in the college program, the prison staff responded by putting them in solitary confinement for thirty days because they thought the men were out of place to mention this learning need. Such is the power of staff at carceral institutions that even framing requests in the wrong way can result in severe penalties and inhumane responses. It is not surprising that Roma's first prison program did not continue beyond two years.

The second choir Roma began in 1993 was UMOJA, the Swahili word for unity. It started in 1994, five years after the Warren Correctional Institution (WCI) opened. But unlike her previous prison program, this choir continued for twenty-three years. This is the longest duration of any outside choral leader shepherding one choir within a US prison that we know of. The role of Warden Anthony Brigano cannot be underestimated: he supported the program and helped lay the foundation for Roma's successful tenure at the prison. It is also highly likely that he mentored the next warden, Wanza Jackson-Mitchell, who continued to support and sustain the program. Key to the leadership they provided was that both of them respected the men in their custody as well as the staff. They created a supportive space for UMOJA and in doing so created the necessary environment for the choir to succeed. The availability of rooms within the facility influenced how educational programming could be scheduled, and with sufficient space for singing together, the men's learning experiences were much improved. WCI was like a college campus, with green spaces the men walked through twice a day as they attended their classes and group programming. The contrast between the physical and managerial aspects of Roma's two choir programs could not be more extreme.

Multiple examples from Roma's choirs illustrate how choral singing can serve as a bridge over prison walls and create spaces to listen to incarcerated Black voices. In the early 2000s, UMOJA performed via telecast in a Martin Luther King program in southwestern Ohio. She began MLK Chorale, co-directing it with Bishop Todd O'Neal for twenty-two years. Rabbi Gary P. Zola suggested they feature UMOJA at the MLK event, and he obtained a grant through AT&T for a live telecast from WCI. Around fourteen UMOJA members sang from the prison infirmary, the only place in the prison with a television connection, normally used for telehealth. Roma was downtown in Cincinnati's Music Hall and connected with the men in the prison on a screen. Lois Shegog, assistant director of MUSE, Cincinnati's Women's Choir, conducted the men inside WCI performing three original pieces by incarcerated Black songwriter Eddie Robertson. The performance was live, and the singers could be seen and heard, but the quality of the sound was fuzzy. Nonetheless, more than 2,000 people in the audience along with people listening to a live radio broadcast in the Music Hall heard primarily Black men's voices from the prison.

Many of the musical experiences discussed so far demonstrate the benefits that outside people bring to those inside a prison. Conversely, musical communities inside prisons can and do support the needs of their local communities. Men in Roma's prison choirs have raised money for charities across Ohio from sales of their four CD recordings, starting in 1997 with *Feel Like Going On*. Roma provided her choir members with a list of several organizations based in the men's home communities. After much discussion, the singers decided to donate to domestic violence shelters, programs to alleviate food insecurity, youth organizations that support system-impacted youth, Murder Victims' Families for Reconciliation, an organization called Cincinnati Cooks that trains and employs formerly incarcerated people as cooks, and a shelter for unhoused people in Wilmington. Representatives from these charities came into WCI to receive cheques from the men in the choir.[5] Roma sent audio and video recordings from the choir to the men's families (Roma 2010). Through Roma's program, incarcerated voices have even garnered international recognition. UMOJA earned two gold medals at the 7th World Choir Games in Cincinnati, Ohio, in 2012, the first time these games were held on the North American continent. Sixty-four countries were represented, with 15,000 participants.[6] Three international judges came inside WCI twice, once to hear the choir perform eight songs in the category of Gospel/Spiritual, and a second time to share the results of the competition with the men. Here, members of UMOJA won gold medals and received international recognition. This was displayed on the world choir games website, in the World Choir Games book, and on YouTube.[7] UMOJA's experience demonstrates that incarcerated voices can communicate beyond prison walls through song, a path of communication resembling that of the prison radio shows in the previous mid-century.[8]

In US state prisons, men can be moved between prisons within any state for many different reasons, such as a change in security category, to complete a required course, for their own safety, to confront disruptive behaviours, or to be closer to family. In 2012, many of UMOJA's members were transferred to London Correctional Institution (LCI). Roma used this moment to start a new men's chorus at LCI, which she named UBUNTU.[9] *Ubuntu* is a Nungni Bantu term that is somewhat difficult to define in Western languages. Desmond Tutu defined *ubuntu* as "my humanity is caught up, is inextricably bound with yours" (Tutu 1999, 31). Five of the men in the UBUNTU Chorus had sung in UMOJA since its inception in 1993, and they helped with the transitional space between the two choirs.

In addition to the challenges facing musical ensembles due to changes in national and state politics and the attitudes of wardens and other prison staff, musical leaders have to manage the challenges that develop when members of the ensemble are suddenly transferred elsewhere. While musical ensembles outside carceral systems, such as town and city choral groups and church choirs, face similar problems, the level of this sort of volatility within the prison system can be much higher depending on the facility.

Since her retirement from academe, Roma has further developed her leadership in ways that support others who want to make positive changes toward dismantling the prison industrial complex. In 2014 she founded Wilmington College's Prison Arts Education Program: the Music, Arts, Theatre Academy (MATA). Its goals are "to build and sustain creative arts offerings in prison. To educate, inspire, motivate, heal and transform lives. To collaborate across fences: inside/outside."[10] She was a founding member of the Ohio Prison Arts Connection (OPAC), a coalition of people from a wide range of backgrounds, including court and corrections personnel, public officials, artists, teachers, funders, and family members who are working to build arts access for people in prisons and to provide re-entry support.[11] MATA and OPAC help sustain Roma's work today, providing opportunities for her programs to grow and develop in new ways.

In 2016, still pursuing new initiatives, Roma founded the KUJI Men's Chorus at Marion Correctional Institution in Marion, Ohio. Kuji is short for *kujichaguila*, which is the second principle of Kwanza, self-determination. Many of the men who sing in KUJI complete a three-day "Growth Potential and Self-Awareness" workshop through the Healing Broken Circles (HBC) program at the facility. HBC's mission is to "provide opportunities to heal, learn, and thrive for those touched by the justice system."[12] This training, according to Roma, has allowed the men in KUJI to manifest the ideas of *ubuntu*.[13]

The Ohio Justice and Policy Center (OJPC), originally the Prison Reform Advocacy Center, commissioned Eddie Robertson to write "Let's Go Make History" for its twentieth anniversary. Robertson, who first sang with UMOJA and joined UBUNTU upon his transfer to LCI, has composed more than sixteen songs. He described "Let's Go Make History" as his all-time favourite (letter to Mary Cohen, December 23, 2019).

> With my heart, with my mind, with my voice
> I have something to say
> Let us reach, for the stars now, when we try, we can go all
>   the way
> There is a light in you, that shines with the light in me
> Together we're burning bright, Let's go make history
> United we can't go wrong, our strength is in unity
> Together we win the fight, Let's go make history.

The UBUNTU Chorus performed it at the OJPC anniversary celebration.[14] The choral performance of "Let's Go Make History" exemplifies how group singing magnifies the lyrical messages performed, generating a broader outlet for social awareness of how much people outside of prison have in common with people in custody. People create a communal body through choral song. In Robertson's lyrics, his use of the plural "we" and his expression that the light that is shining in you is also shining in me illustrates the concept of *ubuntu*. As the chorus expresses this message, the larger communal voice enlivens a sense of *ubuntu*.

Roma's extensive experiences with choral singing and musical community-building over the past three decades have provided opportunities for self-expression for many individuals in prison, created connections between individuals who are incarcerated, and connected people inside and outside of prison, including incarcerated individuals' families, musicians, and other people who hear about her Ohio prison choirs. She has numerous connections with choral communities across Ohio and the US, and through those connections she has broadened awareness of the need for meaningful changes. The complexity of prison issues mandates this kind of intersectional collaboration, a matrix of people from multiple sectors working toward positive transformation.

While Roma's second program is undoubtably a model of success for choral music in prison settings, one worthy of further pedagogical and ethnographical study, her musical ensembles primarily involved incarcerated individuals. We now turn our attention to a different approach to creating musical ensembles, one that brings together incarcerated and nonincarcerated musicians. Upon retirement from a choral conducting career in Anchorage, Alaska, Elvera Voth returned to her home state of Kansas. Through networking at a gathering of Mennonites—a culture known for its social justice initiatives and *a capella* four-part singing at worship—she made connections that allowed her to start a choir at the Lansing Correctional Facility. The minimum-security unit is on the east side of the grounds, hence the name of the choir Voth founded, the East Hill Singers (EHS). To advertise for the choir, Voth had posters placed inside the prison announcing, "Forming a Singing Group," inviting men to join her new prison choir.

Many men thought Voth's choir would be a rap group. About half the men who arrived at that initial rehearsal in 1995 left after the first half, possibly because the style of the choral singing was not what they had anticipated. Perhaps they did not like the lyrics, or perhaps they had other reasons. This high attrition rate signalled to Voth that conscientious attention to musical styles and the message of lyrics are vital for a prison choir facilitator. It is situations like these that highlight the need for culturally relevant and sustaining pedagogies, instructional approaches that had not yet appeared in the literature.

More important than her choices of musical styles were Voth's advocacy of the power of choral singing in broader social contexts and the bringing together of community members and incarcerated men for public performances. Many men at Lansing were new to singing the traditional choral literature in four-part harmony that Voth wanted to introduce to them. She realized they could learn these pieces and develop their vocal sound more effectively if outside volunteer singers joined them. She invited men from the Rainbow Mennonite Church and a few professional singers from the Kansas City Lyric Opera to sing with the choir on concert days. Most members of this outside men's chorus met monthly in Kansas City to rehearse, and eight to ten completed the required Lansing prison volunteer training in order to rehearse once a month with the incarcerated chorus.

With careful oversight by the prison administration, the Lansing men who had no disciplinary infractions were permitted to leave the prison to sing in public concerts with the full outside chorus.[15] On concert days the full EHS chorus would rehearse two hours, take a one-hour break, and then perform for a public audience at 4 p.m. Typically, the choir received warm applause and usually a standing ovation from the audience, and after the performance the incarcerated singers stood in a receiving line to shake hands and receive compliments from audience members. The whole choir would gather after the concert in the church hall for a home-cooked meal. At the first few EHS concerts, prison officers were stationed at every door during performances. Eventually, they sat with the audience, enjoying the concert while completing informal counts of the singers.

Voth had created a powerful model—one ensemble comprised of two very different groups. Both groups gather and sing as one communal voice. This pedagogical approach to blending incarcerated and non-incarcerated singers creates a space for promoting and supporting incarcerated singers' re-entry into society upon release. Research indicates that when people in prison have had positive interactions with volunteers, they are more likely to reintegrate effectively (Duwe and Johnson 2016, 279–303).

The East Hill Singers continued to grow in size, quality, and reputation over the years. Voth, noticing that the men in Lansing craved artistic expression, spearheaded an initiative to provide more arts programming. In doing this she was coming full circle back to her earlier career in Alaska, where in 1968 she had encouraged Robert Shaw to lead the first of his many sing-alongs. Thirty years later, on November 15, 1998, a fundraising Sing-Along with Robert Shaw (1916–99) in North Newton, Kansas, raised $25,000 to start the not-for-profit organization Arts in Prison, Inc. (AiP) (Cohen 2008b).[16] With an executive director and a board of directors, additional programming began.

In graduate school from 2003 to 2007, I (Mary Cohen) assisted with the East Hill Singers, riding regularly with Voth and a few volunteers on the forty-minute drive from Kansas City to Lansing. Occasionally, Voth expressed dissatisfaction with the limited number of additional arts programs in the Lansing prison, even with the AiP not-for-profit organization in place. I began in a new position with AiP as Special Projects Coordinator, recruiting and training outside volunteers to teach in the minimum- and medium-security units in Lansing. These classes included photography, African American history, storytelling, writing, yoga, and visual arts. Besides recruiting and training instructors, we recruited men in the prison to participate. Recruiting incarcerated participants was difficult because communication channels with the men in custody regarding opportunities to participate in the new arts programs were ineffective. Once people began to participate, however, momentum grew. Several individuals said that AiP programs were more meaningful than those required by the DOC. One incarcerated member of the East Hill Singers wrote, "Arts in Prison grows personalities, artistic expression, and individualism" (personal communication).

In the late 1990s, Voth initiated the "West Wall Singers" in Lansing's maximum facility, on the western side of the prison grounds. She recruited local Kansas City music educators Joyce Stuermer and Del Sutton to direct this choir, and the maximum-security chorus thrived for more than eight years. However, the resignation of the two leaders due to health reasons brought this group to an end, demonstrating the challenge of sustainability in such programming, which relies heavily on volunteers and personal charisma. It also demonstrates that without a strong relationship with the warden and staff, it is likely that nothing will be put in place after a musical leader's involvement in a prison comes to an end. Strong relationships with prison staff and a positive community image are clearly important to the long-term sustainability of such programs.

The East Hill Singers concerts have been a source of financial sustainability for AiP. People donate money and purchase art created by AiP students, such as drawings and note cards. But more important than the fundraising, these public events are an opportunity for personal and social transformation. One incarcerated member of the East Hill Singers wrote, "For a few hours I'm an artist, a music lover, a person and not an inmate. This is and always will be priceless." Another indicated that his participation in the EHS was one reason why he was able to reconnect with his sons. His ex-wife decided to bring them to a concert. His performances with the choir allowed his family to see him off drugs and doing something positive. Some men stated that the exuberance of singing together and performing was better than the high they got from drugs. Audience members have transformed their views of men in custody after attending an East Hill Singers concert. One remarked, "For perhaps the first time, the audience was confronted by a group of male prisoners who challenged our stereotypes about them. Here were men singing powerfully about spiritual realities who, regardless of their failures, were undeniably human along with the rest of us" (Waters 1997, 18).

Voth's last performance with the East Hill Singers was at the President's Concert of the Kansas Music Educators' Conference on February 28, 2008.[17] The president of this organization chooses a group to perform for this select spot on the program; traditionally it is a college choir. Some of the audience members were initially shocked when President Jean Ney chose a prison choir for the 2008 President's Concert. But once the music educators in the audience listened to the EHS and heard the choir's message, they encountered a completely new concept: offering music education in a prison setting. This type of attitudinal shift speaks to the significance of broadening purposes and pedagogies in the field of music education. Choral singing has the potential to be a conduit for transformation, but this requires competent, committed, collaborative facilitation that has a clear purpose, keen awareness of what changes are needed, and an instructor with skills in culturally relevant and sustaining pedagogies.

The Kansas Choral Directors Association awarded eighty-four-year-old Voth the "Harry Robert Wilson Award" in July 2008 for all the service she had given to the State of Kansas through her work with EHS and AiP. Many connected to the EHS expressed their deep gratitude. At the June 2008 performance at the Rolling Hills Presbyterian Church in Overland Park, Kansas, the EHS surprised Voth with new lyrics to the song "Elvira," made famous by the Oak Ridge Boys, a US country vocal quartet:

CHORUS
Elvera, Elvera
Our hearts are on fire for Elvera

Eyes that look right through ya
Ears; with pitch so fine
That land can sho nuff make our music shine
We get a funny feeling, deep down in our hearts
When we get it right with singing all four parts

(CHORUS)

She founded Arts in Prison, many years ago
With the East Hill Singers we're sure to put on a show
   (on a show)
Singing all kinds of music
Up and down the scale
And with her guidance we'll just rear back and wail.

(CHORUS)
(last line: *O Elvera, we love you*)

In an interview, Voth noted that one of the things she learned quickly when working with incarcerated men was that "prison life produces men who are tense and wary of expressing themselves" (Waters 1997, 17). Choral singing provides a conduit for self-expression, and with the acknowledgement of the public through audience applause, the experience generates hope and pride. Deputy Warden Allen Ohlstein affirmed, "When the concert audience rose in an overpowering ovation, you could see the pride in the inmates' eyes. Knowing that free-world people respected their efforts seems to have resulted in a valid hope for their futures…something they all too often do not have" (21). Indeed, one of the findings from a research study with this choir is that the men in custody indicated they felt increased self-worth through their participation. Men in the choir also developed a sense of group responsibility, cultivated feelings of accomplishment, and experienced growth in their self-esteem (Cohen 2007b, 66–67). Voth's model of bringing incarcerated and non-incarcerated singers together and performing in public has great potential to broaden social perceptions of people in custody.

Voth's choral model with incarcerated and free voices joining as one community opened my (Mary Cohen's) mind to new purposes for music education. Lansing men were singing side by side with male community volunteers. Some of the Lansing men gave introductions to songs, and audience members congratulated them after the concert. Choral singing provided a passageway to bring two disparate groups together to create a communal voice. Such a communal voice connects individuals through shared vocal expression where people inside and outside prison can listen to incarcerated voices, collaboratively expressing their humanity in an embodied way.

Voth influenced my choice to combine incarcerated and non-incarcerated singers into one choir. In my doctoral studies at the University of Kansas and as a new assistant professor at the University of Iowa, I initiated a research agenda to create a foundational theoretical pedagogy for prison choirs and tested this new theory through research projects. Results of a study that compared well-being measurements between men in a choir and not in a choir indicated significant differences between the two groups on four subscales: sociability, emotional stability, joviality, and happiness. I reached out to other prison choir leaders to learn more about their successes and challenges (Cohen 2009, 319–33; 2012b, 227–34; 2008a) and found that combining incarcerated and non-incarcerated participants held promise for building social awareness about people in custody.

When the Oakdale Community Choir began in 2009, I compared outside volunteers' attitudes toward the incarcerated men in the choir prior to the first rehearsal with their attitudes after the first concert three months later. Outside singers' attitudes toward their fellow singers had improved significantly. Previous stereotypes had been shattered: "I expected them to be in shackles and not interested in singing. I quickly learned that they were human beings, had feelings, and wanted to sing." Another volunteer indicated that people in custody "have taken on personalities instead of being faceless." Comments from incarcerated men highlighted what singing with others, especially with people from outside the prison, meant to them: "The way we were treated ... was like meeting a family I haven't seen for years." One indicated that the choir experience had changed how he viewed other men in the prison, and others noted they were "more outgoing and communicative" and that they had made a lot of friends through singing in the choir. One remarked that he was surprised that after forty years of incarceration, he could "relate to normal people without apprehension" (Cohen 2012a, 51).

In its very first season, the Oakdale Choir initiated a reflective writing exchange among choir members.[18] Its original purpose was to provide an opportunity for choir members to think about what they were singing and share written ideas with one another between Tuesday rehearsals. It also allowed members to build relationships and reflect on ideas. And, it helped me grasp what they thought about singing together and about the songs they were learning. That first choir season, we used Stephen King's 2000 memoir, *On Writing*, as a basis for the writing prompts. Each week, all members received a menu of writing prompts based on King's ideas but applied to singing. We used some of these writings for introductions to the concert selections, shared portions of written reflections at rehearsals, and compiled selections from people's writings in newsletters, sharing those newsletters with the full choir and posting them on the website.[19]

Each semester, we offered a concert for an incarcerated audience, then a second concert for outside guests (plus one choir concert in the summer of 2009). For the first six years, Warden Dan Craig allowed eighty-five outside guests, including family and friends of the choir members, inside the prison gym. Before the concerts we sent messages to all invited guests that described the concert theme and provided information about security and the prison's dress code, instructed them to show deep respect and gratitude to the officers, and informed them about requested arrival times (the schedule had been designed to ease the security process).

A meaningful outcome of the Oakdale Choir was the possibility for incarcerated singers and families to connect in new ways. Inside singers have more topics to discuss. Given the monotony inherent in a prison without programming or educational activities, it can be difficult to think of things to talk about with family members, and this may work against the deepening of relationships. For instance, Richard Winemiller, an inside singer serving a life sentence without parole, described how his relationship with his mother and sister improved through talking about choir, preparing him for a difficult conversation. They were able to discuss his do not resuscitate request calmly (Cohen et al. 2021).

Another inside singer had not had a visit in six years. His family finally decided to drive more than four hours to attend a concert, and since then, he usually has had a guest in the audience on concert days. Given the extreme stress on family dynamics when a member goes to prison, it is important to consider what incarcerated musicians share about their family relationships. Sometimes the crimes they committed were against members of their family, so appropriate attention to support them and their family is vital. Overall, when planning for a prison choir and assessing its growth, family members of incarcerated singers may be able to provide meaningful suggestions and feedback.

On the second day of Warden Jim McKinney's term in October 2015, he came into the room where we were rehearsing. I stopped the current selection, which the group did not know well, and we sang through "Old Irish Blessing," a song more familiar to the choir. It features the text, "May the road rise to meet you, may the wind be always at your back. May the sun shine warm, upon your face, the rains fall soft upon your fields." At the end of that song, Warden McKinney said quietly that that is how he wanted his time at Oakdale to be.

During the same 2015 season, an inside singer used the phrase "Community of Caring" in a written reflection to describe his perception of the choir. It was fitting that the Oakdale Choir used that phrase as its theme during the first season of McKinney's time at Oakdale. The choir's capacity to develop a deep sense of community and care grew tremendously throughout his administrative term. He eventually allowed more than 250 guests into the prison gym for choir events, revealing the extent to which a warden's attitude toward a program impacts its capacity to bridge the divide between incarcerated and free members of society. While McKinney was warden, the choir grew to more than eighty members per season, and more than thirty-five outside singers were allowed to enter the prison to join the inside singers for rehearsals and concerts.

Warden McKinney collaborated with President Bruce Harreld of the University of Iowa to create a new University of Iowa Liberal Arts Beyond Bars (UI LABB) college-credit-bearing program. In this program, faculty came into the prison to teach incarcerated students, who earned college credits. Some classes within the prison included students from the Iowa City campus. The first college-credit-bearing season was in the spring of 2018 and included a choir class with thirty-three men, who earned two hours' college credit for completing "Writing, Singing, and Reflecting in a Choir."[20]

The 2018 and 2019 seasons included several performances outside the prison, although inside singers did not travel outside the prison for these events. On January 16, 2018, on the invitation of Iowa City mayor Jim Throgmorton, I led a surprise choir of outside singers, who sang Melanie DeMore's "Lead with Love" during the community comment period at a meeting of the Iowa City Council.[21] On April 8, 2019, with the invitation or Rep. Mary Mascher, outside members, two former inside members, Warden McKinney, and University of Iowa president Bruce Harreld performed inside the Iowa state capitol in Des Moines.

In May 2018, audio recordings and images of the Oakdale Choir were part of New York–based Heartbeat Opera's production of Beethoven's

Fidelio along with voices and images from five other US prison choirs.[22] In Heartbeat Opera's version of the story, a Black Lives Matter activist was wrongfully convicted. To connect contemporary audiences with the real voices of incarcerated people, six different prison choirs learned and recorded sections of the Prisoners' Chorus, "O welche Lust" (Oh what joy). The company's technical engineers stitched together the audio segments and, in the performance, played the recording of incarcerated voices and showed their images during that portion of the opera. These performances illustrate how the community outside of prison can listen to incarcerated voices through collaborative musical events.

In the fall 2018 season, the Oakdale Community Choir hosted a "Learning Exchange" with the Soweto Gospel Choir from South Africa, Maggie Wheeler (a singer/songwriter and actress who played Janice on the television show "Friends"), and singer/songwriter Sara Thomsen. At this event, rather than identifying groups as "audience" and "performers," everyone was a "participant." We instructed all participants to introduce themselves to one another as they entered the prison gym and settled into their seats. During the event, we sang together, moved together, and spoke with partners related to the theme "Changes We Choose." The event provided opportunities to build social cohesion among participants and dissolved the traditional performer/audience identities that occur in concerts (Harry et al. forthcoming).

In the spring 2019 season, twenty-six students participated in a three-credit-hour UI LABB course, "Peacebuilding, Singing, and Writing in a Prison Choir," in conjunction with singing in the choir. Seventeen of the students were incarcerated, and nine were from the main campus. In addition to class discussions of related readings, the students completed inner peacebuilding projects throughout the semester. In small groups, they developed communal peacebuilding projects, which were displayed on posters at the May 2019 concert, themed "Building Bridges to Peace." Upon approval of this course as a University of Iowa general education requirement in the diversity and inclusion category, in spring 2020, fifteen Iowa City campus students joined fifteen Oakdale campus students for the class and sang in the choir.[23] However, due to the Covid-19 pandemic, the last half of the semester had to be offered virtually, and only five Oakdale students were able to complete the course asynchronously. Warden McKinney retired unexpectedly in May 2020, and the Iowa Department of Corrections stopped all volunteer programming in March 2020 and has not restarted as of summer 2022. Outside singers have become pen pals with inside singers, also supporting former inside singers.

Over ten years, a community of caring has been created between inside and outside choir members. Research investigations, reflections from former incarcerated choir members at concerts and in conversations, informational sharing about re-entry organizations at concerts, and comments from numerous audience members all support our argument that in addition to supporting personal and social growth, choral singing builds social awareness of people in custody. Sung words that relate to the particular experiences of incarcerated individuals provide opportunities for personal and communal reflection. The embodied processes of group singing have both individual and communal outcomes. Some Oakdale Choir audience members have attended concerts consistently, have come to know the inside singers through hearing them perform at concerts, and have checked in with them after concerts about how they and their families are doing. A number of different outlets are continuing to increase this social awareness, including presentations, podcasts, a PBS nine-minute documentary film about the choir, the non-fiction memoir *Redemption Songs: A Year in the Life of a Community Prison Choir* (Douglas 2019), and a documentary film *The Inside Singers* about the choir.[24]

Choral programs in women's prisons address an entirely different need for public awareness. Personal relationships are vital for all people, especially for women behind bars. Choral singing offers a venue for building positive relationships among choir members, musical collaborators, composers, and audiences. Women in prison often experience trauma prior to their incarceration, and they do so more often than men. A study of 100,000 men and women in prisons and jails found that 66 percent of women reported having been diagnosed by a mental health professional, nearly twice the percentage of men. One out of five women and one out of seven men reported recent serious psychological distress (Bronston and Berzofsky 2017). Researchers report the need for gender-responsive programming for women that focuses on building healthy relationships with family and promoting pro-social connections outside of prison (Wright et al. 2012, 1612–32). Social and expressive components of music programs in prisons are especially meaningful and healing for women in custody. Yet very few people have researched, led, or described music education programs in women's prisons. Given all this, the need for research about music education programs for women in custody is vital. In this section, we explore two women's prison choirs: Voices of Hope in the Minnesota Correctional Facility for women at Shakopee, and HOPE Thru Harmony in the Dayton Correctional Institution in Ohio.

In Minnesota, Jim Verhoye, the education director at Shakopee, sought musical leadership for a new choral program he wished to begin. Music faculty at the University of Minnesota saw Verhoye's appeal and suggested to Amanda Weber, a choral conducting graduate student, that she consider this opportunity. Verhoye and Weber got together and launched this project, which began as a series of twelve-week classes in the prison's education department. On October 14, 2015, Amanda Weber started Voices of Hope (VOH) with seventeen singers within the prison.

To develop a mission statement grounded in all members' experiences with the choir, Weber invited each singer to write a response to the question "Why do you sing?" She identified three categories in their responses: self, ensemble, and wider community. From an analysis of these individual statements, the following mission was crafted: "The

Voices of Hope is a women's prison choir that fosters individual growth and bridges unlikely communities through song." It also declared the following goals:

> (1) BRINGING HOPE TO MINNESOTA CORRECTIONAL FACILITY-SHAKOPEE: The Voices of Hope provides a safe and sober activity which empowers women to find their voice, build connections in a diverse setting, and bring a positive message of hope and healing to the MCF-Shakopee community. (2) BRINGING HOPE OUTSIDE PRISON WALLS: The Voices of Hope views singing as a powerful tool of restorative justice, seeking to transform perspectives of incarceration and build bridges of healing within the wider community through collaboration and reflection. (Weber 2018, 80)

Weber's process of crafting a mission statement based on her singers' reflections has its roots in the restorative principles of accomplishing things *with* rather than *for* or *to* others. Such an approach provides a sense of group ownership and communal identity among members of the choir and inspires investment in its future. In contrast to prevalent approaches within US criminal legal systems, rather than asking who committed a crime and how it should be punished, restorative principles centre around questions related to responsivity: Who has been hurt, what are their needs, and whose obligations are these? This concept of wrongdoing is based on the understanding that we are all interconnected (Zehr 2002, 19–22).

Creating interconnectedness can be difficult for music leaders in prisons, for they must navigate the physical and social separations that are foundational to prison life. Music leaders coming into facilities on a weekly basis have only a finite amount of time to connect with learners. Furthermore, in Voices of Hope, most members sing in the choir for only one quarter (or twelve weeks). Relationships among members and a sense of group identity need to be rebuilt each choir season. Weber noted that within the sacred space of choir, the members of VOH work to create a space that is countercultural to the prison setting. Additionally, participants new to singing need to learn basic vocal techniques in addition to the songs. For the women in Shakopee, the average length of sentence is fifty-six months (excluding life sentences). As of January 2022, 278 women have sung in the Voices of Hope Choir, and 247 of them (89%) have been released from prison (personal correspondence, January 5, 2022).

VOH has developed into a consistent choir through regular twelve-week sessions. Over the first three years, it grew to more than fifty members. Weber's choir has become a special group within Shakopee and has developed a communal identity. She purposefully started small when bringing additional singers into the prison, first by developing collaborative workshops with a women's choir from the University of Minnesota. Members of that choir learned some of the same songs as VOH and then came inside the prison to spend time with each other, deepening their relationships, and to sing together. During the 2016–17 academic year, this collaborative workshop model expanded into a project called Phenomenal Woman. Inspired by Maya Angelou, the project included compositions and texts by women, including four of Angelou's poems. The theme celebrated who they are and led to commissions for a text, "O Sister," by University of Minnesota poet D. Allen, who created lyrics based on words and phrases from the VOH members. Canadian composer Kathleen Allan then composed a choral arrangement with these lyrics.

Jim Verhoye encouraged Weber to facilitate interactions between those outside and those inside the prison: "The more we bring the community into the prison, the more the prison becomes more like the community in a good way" (Weber 2018, 218). Weber chose to include outside participants for special projects rather than having them sing consistently with the choir, a choice that eased the burden on prison staff. Without seasoned singers as a regular part of the choir, members of VOH have become more independent music leaders than they might otherwise have been. Weber reports that they find value in developing musical and vocal skills without outside help.

Many women in prison have experienced trauma at the hands of men (McDaniels-Wilson and Belknap 2008, 1090–127), and in their daily lives they are subject to male as well as female voices of authority. Weber described the experience of sixty outside singers, including men, as they joined the women to perform "Shenandoah." When the arrangement began with the men singing in unison softly, Weber noticed, "one by one, every single woman in Voices of Hope began crying" (116). The unexpected experience of men singing in a caring and beautiful way was deeply emotional for them.

Depending on the particular collaboration this choir is doing, VOH may have male, female, or both male and female outside singer volunteers. According to Weber, women develop pride through their practice of hospitality in the choir, which is what community music scholar Lee Higgins delineates as gestures of welcoming, invitations to be included, and unconditional acceptance (Higgins 2012, 133–43). These acts of hospitality, which are made to volunteers regardless of gender, bring about positive changes among those who enter the prison to sing with them. One outside volunteer, Bill Gurnon, described his personal transformation after two months of singing with VOH in his book *Three O'Clock Movement: Revelation in a Women's Prison*. He noted that his implicit bias against people in prison stemmed from watching episodes of *Gunsmoke* more than sixty years prior, when he was only nine years old. That TV show, which ran from 1955 to 1975, centred on Marshal Dillon of Dodge City, Kansas, who captured the "bad guys" and put them in jail to teach them a lesson. Gurnon described how he loved *Gunsmoke* "despite (or maybe because of) its simplistic approach to justice" (Gurnon 2018, 13).

Sixty years later, he accepted an invitation to sing with VOH because he loved singing in choirs, was intrigued by the idea of outsiders joining a prison choir, and he knew and admired Weber's skills as a choral director. His initial intentions for joining did not include learning about incarcerated women or considering problems or policies related to prisons. During the volunteer training, he went on a tour of the prison and was shocked that it had large green plants, a small chapel, a gymnasium, and a library. Outside, he saw volleyball courts, walking paths, flower gardens, and a picnic area. Even so, during the week between the volunteer training and his first choir rehearsal with VOH, he assumed that the women would be tough and dangerous, with hostile and angry attitudes.

He had ambivalent feelings about meeting them and being with them for ninety minutes each Sunday afternoon. Then he met them. Fifty women were excited and happy to sing with this choir. He sat between Jessica and Natalie and shared a belief with Jessica that life existed on other planets and learned that Natalie wanted to start a support group for battered women when she was released. Gurnon felt honoured to sing with them and was surprised how he enjoyed being around them. Rehearsals were powerful opportunities for the women to share their stories. He heard stories of choir members who were afraid to be released for fear of a partner beating or raping them. Through his experiences in this choir, he began to realize that he had been biased against people in prison; he no longer believed the myth that people are either good or bad. He had never questioned his beliefs about people in prison prior to singing in VOH. His mistaken views had been "hiding in the shadows of prejudice. In many ways, they were impenetrable" until he began singing with them (47).

The Phenomenal Woman concert was offered only to incarcerated women inside Shakopee. The women did not have approval to perform outside the facility. So a decision was made to perform this concert outside the prison, in Minneapolis, on February 24, 2017, with only outside choristers. In solidarity with the women of VOH, the outside chorus members wore pink choir T-shirts, and as a reminder of the women they displayed the blue Voices of Hope T-shirts that the inside women wear for performances. In one song, they used an audio recording of VOH that seamlessly shifted into the women's chorus voices. Such innovative and purposeful programming visually and audibly symbolized the missing bodies of VOH members and provided audiences with a clear portrayal of the women's voices. Through this weaving together, the audience members were able to listen to the women's voices even though they were not physically present. During the performance, the choristers surrounded the audience and spoke the name of each VOH singer as another way to bring them all into the room.

A student from the women's chorus reflected on the growth she experienced by collaborating with VOH: "My love of music was a selfish love. I craved the look of amazement on people's faces when they heard me sing. I needed to perform and sing louder and higher than everyone around me." After singing with VOH and performing with them in the Phenomenal Woman concert, she "realized music's true purpose. It is not about self-promotion. It is salvation...Until seeing the unimaginable strength and power of the Voices of Hope, I was blind. Their singing saved me" (77). These concerts have inspired family members of VOH singers to speak out about the criminal legal system. One VOH member described how her mother encouraged people to attend the collaborative concerts and how this prompted conversations about incarceration (137). In these ways, the women's communal voice became a channel for deeper understanding of injustices related to prisons and the criminal legal system.

Weber's responsibilities include weekly choir director duties and community-building activities through collaborative projects with people outside the prison (107). In her weekly choir director duties, she has created a sense of ritual in her classroom: similar chair set-up each week, warm-ups at the beginning of practices, traditions marking the start and end of each quarter. This consistency allows singers who have sung for one quarter with VOH to step into leadership positions to support new members. Weber suggests that this development of a communal mind-set provides a "resistance to the survival setting of a prison" (104).

In May 2017, Weber took steps to start a not-for-profit, with fiscal sponsorship from Springboard for the Arts, an economic and community development organization based in St. Paul (72). She has received musical and organizational support from the leadership team created to support the choir. That team continues to evolve, and primarily includes circles of support with three college interns and three choral mentors. She sometimes refers to this group as the choir's "volunteer team," as only their accompanist and vocal coach are paid. They have a part-time executive director; Weber's official title is founder and artistic director. VOH has performed twice each year at prison graduation ceremonies and for audiences of up to one hundred incarcerated women. With the addition of around fifteen outside guests to collaborate with the singers for these events, they have made a step toward meeting Verhoye's goal of bringing outside community members into the prison.

Weber has created a space in Shakopee where the women bravely find their voices, take steps toward healing, and feel empowered in the process. Her mindful choice of incorporating outside volunteers only for specific projects gives the women more autonomy, allows them to practise hospitality, and provides incremental steps toward building more positive relationships with men through increased social awareness.

Before leading prison choirs, Catherine Roma's choral scholarship centred on creating women's choirs, empowering women to seek equal pay, developing effective health care, and supporting the rights of people who are part of the LGBTQA+ community. When creating a women's prison choir, she continued these aims. After retiring from Wilmington College in 2014, while leading the two men's prison choruses described earlier in this chapter, Roma founded HOPE Thru Harmony Women's Choir at the Dayton Correctional Institution (DCI) in Ohio. She began with twenty-two singers from inside the facility and seven to fourteen singers from Cincinnati, Middletown, Dayton, and Yellow Springs.

They dedicated their initial concert, themed "Lift Me Up to the Light of Change," to Wanza Jackson-Mitchell, who served as warden of DCI from December 2014 through early 2018. This concert included literature that speaks about women's lives. One singer, Megan, described her experience with the performance in a way that highlights the word and somatic factors: "I had the honor to participate in the singing and poetry. It was so empowering to see how the words, melodies, movements all flowed together to captivate the entire room of people. I felt we were all connected—that each song—each word—each tone slowly intertwined our feelings, our lives, our souls so that by the time we closed the final notes, the room was one, we were united in common experience, common humanity, and it was breath taking" (MATA n.d.). Choral singing was a powerful embodied experience that enabled these women to connect with one another and the audience through words, human expression, and song.

Warden Jackson-Mitchell created a supportive environment in the prison. The women had opportunities to participate in a variety of arts and educational programs including art therapy, college classes, a program called Women Empowering Women, and many special musical events that Roma facilitated. These events included musical guest composer Ysaye Marie Barnwell, who visited the prison twice. In her first visit she led a workshop on a few of her compositions, including "We Are." At that workshop she told them about "Crossings," her five-movement piece for chorus, narrator, and dancers. The pieces include: "Uptown Overture," "No Mirrors in My Nana's House," "Lost in Blue," "When I Die," and "Wanting Memories." They decided on the spot to learn this *a capella* song suite.

Barnwell's second visit, on Saturday, July 14, 2017, was to hear HOPE Thru Harmony's performance of "Crossings." The women's chorus included college students from Earlham College and professional women from the community. She raved about the performance, noting that the interchange between women in custody, working women, and college students had been "magical." She suggested that the performance should be videotaped because the "students need to see themselves being in relationship with those whose experiences they can hardly begin to understand" (Ysaye Barnwell, email to Catherine Roma, July 14, 2017). Alphonse Gerhardstein, a civil rights attorney and founder of the Ohio Justice and Policy Center, who was also at the performance, sent a strong letter of support to the director of the Ohio Department of Corrections, stating:

> There is something different about a few residents getting together to "sing" and this choral group mastering the profound and moving works we heard on Saturday. I could see the residents beaming and standing proud as they took their bows, as they congratulated the solos among them, as they performed so well under pressure. You have in Dr. Cathy Roma and her colleagues rare leaders who have gained the trust of these residents. These performers were not cut any slack. They were excellent on every objective level. I suspect that this choral experience is for many a first encounter with total success in such a challenging and rewarding enterprise…Thanks for facilitating this choral program and I hope more like it can be developed. (email to Catherine Roma, April 14, 2017)

Roma and HOPE Thru Harmony have collaborated with MUSE Cincinnati Women's Choir led by Jillian Harrison-Jones, with commissioned composer Rosephanye Powell, with the Earlham College Women's Ensemble led by Danielle Cozart Steele, and with University of Chicago choral conductor Mollie Stone.[25] Powell and Stone have led workshops with the HOPE Thru Harmony singers, further developing their vocal and musical skills.

Roma carefully chooses the choral literature for incarcerated women. These compositions have included a combined arrangement of

"True Colors" by Robert Hazard and "Ooo Child (Things Are Gonna Get Easier)" by Stan Vincent, "Listen to the Voices" by Holly Near, "And She Will Rise" by Dakota Butterfield, "Breaths" by Brago Diop, "Blessing" by Joan Szymko, and "Circle Chant" by Linda Hirshhorn.

Tenor John Wesley Wright has visited Roma's prison choirs and describes how choral experiences for incarcerated women provide a space for them to feel, trust, and show emotion, as well as speak constructively to one another (Wright 2019, 573–77). HOPE Thru Harmony has given two performances for families where outside volunteers brought in homemade food. These caring experiences were healing for all involved and created positive memories for families. This environment also created a space for leaders to emerge within the prison choir.

In 2015, Roma collaborated with Emily Steinmetz, a professor of anthropology at Antioch College, in a mini-course at DCI called "Women, Leadership, and Community Empowerment." Four Antioch College juniors and Roma created a six-week writing and reading class where the women's pieces were collected into a "zine." Roma's leadership has provided educational programming for women at DCI that they otherwise would not have had.

After Jackson-Mitchell left DCI, the atmosphere in the prison changed. Fewer programs were available, and the new administration placed restrictions on what Roma could offer the women in HOPE Thru Harmony. Still, she continued to develop the choir as best she could. The warden's approach toward programming has strongly impacted what the choral singing program can accomplish at DCI.

This testimonial from a HOPE Thru Harmony choir member reveals some of the potential of choral singing in prisons: "I've been incarcerated for almost twelve years and last Saturday was the first time I felt closest to home. All of my friends and family were there to support with tears, laughter, and awe. It was so familiar and welcomed" (MATA n.d.).

In Ohio, as in other states, incarcerated women do not receive the same types of resources as are available to men. Moreover, as Roma notes, women are not given the same type and number of responsibilities as are offered to men. In men's prisons, men are given leadership roles in the functioning of the facility, but in Roma's experience, women have not been empowered with such leadership tasks. As noted earlier, many women in prison have been traumatized by men, so male officers in women's prisons can be highly distressing for some women. Research indicates that the risk and need factors for women in prison are different from those men face. Without effective training for all prison staff to learn how to interact with women experiencing trauma, and without effective programming, women are left on their own to figure out how to navigate their difficult experiences.

In this chapter, we have described how choral singing, through its embodied experiences and sung words, provides a powerful space for people in custody to develop a sense of self-worth and confidence, as well as to express themselves and connect with others. Relationships among singers are built through the creation of a communal vocal body. When community members, including families and friends of people in custody, can attend choral performances, the ensuing social growth leads to increasing social awareness of the humanity of people behind bars. Additionally, the sung words have the potential to broaden social awareness through impactful messages related to a choir's purpose. When those words are created by the people in custody, even more impactful and more productive outcomes are possible. We explore this in the next chapter, about songwriting in prisons.

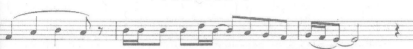

CHAPTER 5

"LIFE WITHIN THESE WALLS"

The Dynamic and Interactive Nature of Songwriting in Prisons

*C*reating and performing original songs has many personal and social benefits to offer incarcerated populations. It can also broaden society's awareness of the humanity of people behind bars. When a choir performs an original song composed by a member, and that individual receives affirmation from peers and audience members, such personal expression builds the songwriter's sense of worthiness and competence. When audience members listen to feelings and experiences through performances of original songs, they may begin to develop a deeper and more intimate connection to the songwriter, and if that songwriter is incarcerated, greater social awareness of people in custody is possible.[1] However, prisons are often difficult environments to achieve these outcomes.

In prisons, socially acceptable opportunities for shared self-expression are limited. Prison units are designed and managed in ways that minimize group engagement. People in custody have limited outlets for healthy personal and communal self-expression. Individuals are required to wear a uniform and are assigned a number, stripping them of part of their individuality, for they are not called by their first name, but rather by a number or their last name. Music-making within prisons is restricted by limited access to musical instruments, controlled access to space for musical practice, and rules about how many incarcerated individuals can gather for rehearsals. From our examination of a wide variety of songwriting programs and our research on songwriting in a men's prison, it is clear that when incarcerated individuals have access to the means to create original lyrics and songs, they are able to process difficult emotions, reflect on their life journeys, communicate feelings for family members, and share personal stories, metaphors, and humour (Bulgren 2020, 299–318; Cohen and Wilson 2017, 543–51; Wilson 2013).

Collaborative songwriting projects can be difficult to develop in a prison environment, given the power dynamics and the wide range of musical backgrounds among both incarcerated and non-incarcerated participants. Songwriting involves the creative processes of writing lyrics and creating musical settings to accompany those lyrics; these can be done separately or simultaneously. In the Oakdale Prison Songwriting Workshops, sometimes one individual creates the entire song, sometimes a collaborative partnership or small group works to write a song together, sometimes an entire choir is involved in the songwriting process, and sometimes one person writes lyrics and another sets them to music (Cohen and Wilson 2017). In this chapter, when we refer to songwriting, we are referring to any of these possibilities, and we explore the intricate power dynamics related to songwriting processes.

The Oakdale Prison Summer Songwriting Workshops began as a result of incarcerated singers' prolific self-expression in lyric-writing and as an extension of the reflective writing exchange. The Liz Lerman

Critical Response Process, a four-step, strength-based feedback process (Lerman and Borstel 2003), provided a framework for Oakdale songwriters to discuss the lyrics and songs as they evolved. This process generated dialogues about songwriting. At times, the sometimes quite personal topics shared in original lyrics were a core part of songwriting experiences.

In the academic literature, songwriting falls mainly under the umbrella of music therapy or popular music education pedagogy. The purpose of songwriting in prisons is not to create bestselling songs, though some people in custody may dream of writing a bestselling song and acquiring fame and wealth. Some programs, such as Jail Guitar Doors, address this desire directly, explaining how difficult the music industry is.[2] Pedagogically, the goals include expressing oneself through songwriting, creating material for a choir or others to sing, offering a space for giving and receiving positive and constructive feedback, and providing a venue for discussing ideas expressed in original songs. Additionally, songwriting offers opportunities for personal and social growth and builds social awareness in more intimate ways than musical performances of compositions written by people who have no connection to the prison ensemble.

In addition to all this, the co-creation processes possible with choral singing and songwriting generate social growth in ways that other forms of music-making do not. Birthing an original song for performance with a full choir is a communal experience to which all members contribute. As a choir rehearses a new song, the group can try different choices in the structure, melody, rhythms, harmonies, and lyrics and notice how these changes impact the song's feeling and message; in this way, all members play a role in creating the choral arrangement of the original song. What was once a spark of an idea inside one incarcerated person's heart becomes embodied in a group of singers and heard by an audience of listeners. When this occurs, the members of a choir build a special communal identity in their shared experience of developing, learning, and performing an original song, as well as a unique connection with their fellow choir member who wrote the song.

In a choir setting, observational feedback from choir members can transform an incarcerated songwriter's self-concept. Lyrics are an important consideration when deciding which songs a choir will sing. In the first season of the Oakdale Choir, the focus was on lyrics, which left out considerations of other musical elements such as tempo. Many of the songs selected for that first performance were slow and sentimental.[3] Incarcerated choir member Kenneth Bailey heard a comment I made to the choir about this, and toward the end of the first season, he wrote a set of lyrics titled "Crossroads." They had an upbeat message about moving on with life.[4] Prior to writing these lyrics, he had shared some of his original poetry, which conveyed very dark messages. The titles of these poems were "Hell's Flames," "Bone Orchard," and "Apollo's Conquest."

In the second Oakdale Choir season, rather than engaging in a reflective writing exchange with prompts based on a book,[5] the writing prompts invited members to craft lyrics for new songs. Some of the men wrote music with their lyrics, others created lyrics and asked me to set them to music. One of the lyrics I set to music was Kenneth's "Crossroads." Kenneth told me it had taken him a lot of courage to share these lyrics with me, and the day he did, before quickly leaving the room, he told me I could set them to music any way I wished. The week after the "Rivers and Rocks" August 2009 concert where we premiered "Crossroads," Kenneth reflected that after hearing the outside singers repeatedly tell him how much they liked "Crossroads," he realized that his original lyrics and poems had been transformed—they were now lighter and more upbeat. This man, who had gained forty pounds in his first six months of incarceration and who had intended to "do his time alone," had undergone a profound change through singing in the choir: he had expressed himself through original lyrics and found the courage share them with others. He continued to build his creativity by participating in the songwriting workshop and a writers' workshop and by creating many original lyrics, including a song Yo-Yo Ma would later perform.[6]

Original songs also provide seeds for connections across prison barriers, as our next story illustrates. Before starting with the Oakdale Summer Songwriting Workshop, Kenneth sketched his musical ideas for a song called "May the Stars Remember Your Name" on a sheet of lined notebook paper with a hand-drawn musical staff. He wrote this song in the hope that he would one day be released from prison and again be able to see the stars, which he could not during his incarceration because of the bright security lights that erased the stars from the sky. The metre on his handwritten score was triple, and he had a general idea written out for the shape of the melody. I took his idea to my piano and developed the song, then brought a draft of it to the prison to share with him. He liked the creation, and we performed it in the spring 2010 concert themed "More Love."

Meade Palidofsky, founder of Storycatchers Theater in Chicago,[7] came to the dress rehearsal for this concert and asked permission to use the song with her Fabulous Females program at the Illinois Youth Center at Warrenville. They adapted Kenneth's song for their fall original musical, "Mom in the Moon." Because Storycatchers has a partnership with the Chicago Symphony Orchestra (CSO), Riccardo Muti, director of the CSO, came to Warrenville (WYC) to listen to the youth perform their adaption of Kenneth's "May the Stars Remember Your Name." Through this partnership, a string arrangement of Kenneth's song was created, and Yo-Yo Ma came to WYC in October 2010 to perform this arrangement with a group of musicians from the CSO. I attended this performance and shared the story of the Oakdale Choir, Kenneth's song, and Palidofsky's visit to Iowa. Yo-Yo Ma complimented this project and emphasized how collaboration is necessary for such amazing things to happen (Cohen 2019a, 142–45).

Audiences of the Oakdale Community Choir have regularly reported how meaningful it is for them to hear original songs performed by the choir. One audience member wrote, "I am compelled to articulate how much human connectivity resonated throughout the concert and what it meant for the inside choir members to share their lives, and their truth. To experience the weaving of lives into an expression of music was an emotional overflow for me, a positive emotional experience I'll never forget." This experience of listening to original songs written by incarcerated individuals and performed by a choir of incarcerated and community members deepened this individual's insight into the humanity of the men in custody. This "positive emotional experience" combined many elements: it fostered incarcerated individuals' creative thoughts through song; it combined those personal expressions into one communal voice; and it shared them with guests, some of whom were their families. Perhaps part of what was meaningful for audience members was the raw difficulties expressed through some of the original songs.

The challenging experiences expressed through original songs from Oakdale Choir members include relationship problems, missing others, regret, pain, needing help, and issues with living in prison (Cohen and Wilson 2017). One of many difficulties of songwriting in prisons is the need to balance delicate egos with healthy affirmations. One inside Oakdale Choir member warned of these issues during the first season of the choir:

> The biggest downside to the choir, as far as I'm, concerned, is that I see men who are in prison basically because of behaviours dictated by overinflated egos continue to feed their self-centredness. I see this because it is something that I have to combat in myself. How do you balance efforts to lift up self-esteem against the possibility of enabling a person to stay stuck in a narcissistic delusional world where the wants and needs of others are always subservient or non-existent? Encouraging someone to step up and perform may be forcing them out of a shell of shyness or self-pity. It may

also, in his mind, validate his belief that he is better than those around him. It's a swampy mess that I think needs to be in the back of our minds. (Cohen 2012a)

Without any counselling support or some other professional healing outlet for choir members, and without a mechanism to listen to the needs and feelings of choir members, some group singing experiences of original songs could cause unintended harm. For example, the week after the Oakdale Choir first practised Kenneth Bailey's song, "Crossroads," Davis Anderson gave me a handwritten set of lyrics to "In My Mother's Eyes" and asked me to set it to music. When I arrived home and read through the lyrics, I was moved by his message. He wrote the song as a reflection on the look his mother gave him when he was sentenced to prison and as an expression of his craving for the look of care and love she used to give him, the look that "keeps the dreams away at night." I carefully selected metre in three, like a lullaby, and D minor tonality to depict a feeling of sadness and longing, then brought a draft of the song to a choir rehearsal. After the first run-through, I turned toward the choir from the piano and saw one inside singer taking his glasses off to wipe tears from his eyes. Everyone clapped immediately after the song was over. Then another inside singer said, "That was the most beautiful thing I have heard since I have been in prison." After a long pause, the choir members shared how they could all relate to disappointing a parent and knew how challenging it is for incarcerated individuals to face a parent in the wake of being sentenced to prison.

Two seasons later, I reintroduced "In My Mother's Eyes" with a new arrangement of the chorus in four-part harmony. In the meantime, many people had spoken positively to Davis about his song. Kevin B.F. Burt, a professional blues musician, talked about using his song. I found out later that all these experiences fed Davis's ego in a way that irritated the other inside singers. I received an anonymous typed note:

Dr. Cohen, I am writing this letter to bring a problem to your attention. I as well as several other offenders are really tired of the song, "In My Mother's Eyes." Yes, the song has meaning, but, as offenders, we do not need to have this type of song run in the ground as this one has here at IMCC. A few offenders have considered dropping out of the choir after this song was passed out last week and, one will on March 2, partially due to this song.

Out of our hearts, please select a different score as we know there are many worthy of their time (Scores). The hype given to this song has created a monster and ill feelings with the offenders. Thank you.

We dropped the song "In My Mother's Eyes" that season, and the choir did not perform it again. The social interactions surrounding the song had negatively impacted Davis's relationship with the other inside singers. And the content of the song may have reintroduced trauma about being sentenced to prison. Additionally, my role as outside leader of the group carried a power dynamic that I had used ineffectively when I decided to reintroduce Davis's song without discussing this idea with the choir members.

As outside instructors for songwriting in prisons, it is difficult for us to understand the types of stresses people in custody experience. Songwriting can be a means to express all sorts of feelings, and the process can be a tool for enhancing awareness of one's emotions and for building communication skills. Such outlets are more effective when someone guides and supports songwriters. For example, at the Marmot High School inside the Youth Correctional Center in Mandan, North Dakota, one of Megan Holkup's students who only had one month in class before release had a goal of writing lyrics to one song. He apologized to Ms. Holkup for how dark his lyrics were. Holkup encouraged him by explaining how writing descriptions of what one is going through can build an emotional vocabulary to describe feelings and acknowledge one's circumstances more effectively. This conversation compelled him to record his song, share it with someone else, and then write and record seven additional songs. His process of creating songs allowed him to acknowledge his triggers, such as grief. His last few pieces expressed hope, plans for his future, and eventually a song about having a good time. He reflected that "These rhymes … they save my life" (Megan Holkup, email to Mary Cohen, November 21, 2018). Songwriting instruction, facilitated with a deeply caring attitude, created the opportunity for this student to build the self-efficacy he needed to generate the will to live.

The students at Marmot created graduation compositions, and in 2018 they received permission to make a YouTube video titled "Road to Glory." Eleven students wrote the lyrics, noting that their words were "for everyone who is struggling … not just us." An excerpt from their lyrics:

> Need to overcome the dark and find the light
> I gotta keep my head high if I want to have my future bright
> The further I get the more I stumble
> Get back up and refuse to crumble
> Even though I make mistakes I know I'll go far
> Even though the road to success is hard
> I can be the shining star
> This is the hand I was dealt
> I'm just playing the cards.[8]

These students had created a shared reflection on their difficult life experiences. The lyrics reflect that they had taken ownership of their past mistakes.

In this instance, group songwriting provided a space for the students to be resilient and hopeful despite the difficulties they had faced. Holkup's affirming teaching approach supported the learners individually and collectively, guiding them toward a hopeful future.

The students' experiences of expressing themselves musically and collaborating on a music video generated trust and developed their teamwork skills. When songwriters feel empowered to honour their feelings as they create original songs and lyrics, catharsis and a sense of release allow deeper personal growth. Group work with songwriting and producing a video provides opportunities for social growth. With permission from the facility to share the video on YouTube, the musical creation became a means for the youth to share their group composition beyond the facility and for society to listen to incarcerated voices.

In addition to youth who are in custody, who directly experience trauma from incarceration, more than 5.7 million children in the US—that is, one in every twelve youth under eighteen—experience the stress and stigma of having a parent in prison (Gotsch 2018, 7). The tearing apart of families through incarceration is extremely painful to those who experience it, and songwriting is a means for incarcerated parents to express their feelings about it.[9]

Patrick Wilson, an inside Oakdale singer, wrote "To My Daughter Erica Linnette" for his baby daughter, who was born two months and eleven days after his incarceration. He had not yet held her or even met her. In his song he conveyed his love for Erica and asked for her forgiveness. Patrick introduced his song to an outside audience, and this experience touched their hearts in ways they had not anticipated.

> So little and so sweet
> Never have I met you
> Not that I don't want to
> I may not be there
> But in my dreams, I'm with you
> And we have time to share
> I just want you to know
> That you hold all my love.

The bridge of Patrick's song expresses his plea for forgiveness, his acknowledgement of his selfish actions, and his deep yearning to be with his family:

> You are my little girl and I want to be there
> You are my little girl, and I want you to know that I really
>   do care
> I'm sorry I've been gone for so long
> I'll admit I was acting selfish all along
> But now I need my family with me more than anyone
>   would believe.

University of Iowa students enrolled in a human rights class attended the concert where Patrick's song was premiered, and they described how extremely emotional his song was and how they hoped Patrick would be reunited with his family. Those who attended the concert or listened to the recording heard Patrick's deep personal difficulties of being separated from his baby daughter and his family.

Varrus Valor, an Oakdale Choir member and songwriting participant, wrote "Missing for So Long" for his two sons to tell them how much he missed them and to apologize for not being around during their formative years:

> 1. You reached for my hand, it wasn't there
>   It's been missing for years
>   One day it was there, to help soothe away your fears
>   The next it wasn't and I let you fall, and I'm sorry that
>
>   CHORUS
>   *My guiding hand can't help you along*
>   *It's been bound and hidden, missing for so long*
>   *Gone and not there, you need to be strong*
>   *To not lose hope, and hope it's not long.*

2. I wrote you a letter the other day
   Cause you're on my mind
   I wish I was there to help you when you fall down
   I'm sorry I won't be there till you're a man
   That was not my plan

FINAL CHORUS

My guiding hand is praying for you now
It may seem bound and hidden, missing for so long
Gone and not there, you need to be strong
To not lose hope & hope it's not long.
I pray it's not too long.[10]

Varrus's song revealed a longing and sadness that many of the other men in the prison were experiencing. Much like Patrick's, Varrus's lyrics expressed the personal difficulties he had faced as a parent in prison unable to be with his children.

Sometimes original songs express love for family members who have died. Grieving can be understood as the private expression of coming to terms with the death of a close relation. Mourning can be understood as a public expression of one's grief. Both are vital for anyone dealing with death and loss in their lives. For people in custody, opportunities to express bereavement are extremely limited. The rules for whether a person in custody can attend a family member's funeral vary depending on a host of issues, including the relationship of the family member to the person in custody, the location of the funeral, whether the person in custody has had any recent disciplinary reports, and the discretion of the prison supervisors.

When someone in custody cannot attend a funeral or needs to process emotions related to grief, songwriting can serve as a meaningful outlet. For example, charter Oakdale Choir member and songwriter Kenneth Bailey wrote the lyrics to "Watching Over Me" in memory of his great-grandmother, "Gram," whom he described as one of the most remarkable human beings he was blessed to know. During some of the rehearsals, he conducted the choir as they practised his song. Every time he did, emotions swarmed over him at the memories that bubbled up through hearing the song. Kenneth expressed solace in knowing that Gram never left him; she continued to watch over him. Some of the lyrics to the song:

> I'm listening for you as the rain falls from up above,
> I'm searching 'cross the skies so I can see what you've become,

> CHORUS
> *Because I feel you, around every corner,*
> *I feel you as my day is growing warmer,*
> *And I miss you, Oh, I miss you,*
> *'Til I smile once again, and I know you are there,*
> *Watching, Watching Over Me.*

Catherine Wilson, who at the time was a doctoral student in music education, set Kenneth's lyrics to music. With Kenneth's and Wilson's permission, my family used this song at my sister Judy's funeral. Judy died unexpectedly the Sunday before the final choir rehearsal of the spring 2012 season. One week after her death, Judy's friends hosted a celebration of her life. At this event they gave orange stretchy bracelets that read "WWJudyD?" (What Would Judy Do?) with the answer "Find the Joy." As part of the grieving process, I wrote lyrics and music to an original song, "Find the Joy." I explored the question: How do we find joy when we are living through grief? During the spring 2013 semester, the Oakdale Choir learned this song for the themed concert "Mourning Is Broken." The lyrics begin:

> How can I find the joy when brick walls block my path?
> How can I find the joy when I'm living through the aftermath?

CHORUS
Oh, where is the joy? Where is the joy?
Where is the joy? I'm looking for the joy.

The experience of bringing this song to life through the communal voice of the Oakdale Choir, and sharing it with an audience, was a deeply healing experience for me. As the choir was learning the song, members checked in with me to inquire how I was navigating the grief. One of the outside singers, Kevin Kummer, shared with me that in his experience, joy is not something outside of ourselves that we need to go out to find. Rather, it is always within us. With this new insight, I changed the final lyrics of the song to: "*We pause and feel the joy.*"

The process of bringing "Find the Joy" and "Watching Over Me" to life provided both personal growth and an opportunity to mourn publicly through performing in the prison and sharing audio recordings. An extreme amount of loss and grief occurs through incarceration. Johnathan Kana, a formerly incarcerated songwriter from Texas, wrote in his song "Life within These Walls" how people in prison experience a metaphorical death. One inside Oakdale Choir member reflected on a lyrical line in "Death by Institution" by observing that imprisonment often amounts to a death of expectations for one's future:

> To me it means disoriented and confused institution that struggles to find a remedy for the recovery of sons, fathers, grandfathers, and husbands from their society. Death is everywhere in these walls filled with questions and expectations for a tomorrow that may not come for a prisoner.

Songwriting, singing original songs, and reflecting upon their messages can serve as a natural outlet for expressing and working through grief, pain, and trauma. These stories illustrate how songwriting may create an opportunity to share feelings through original songs, to develop empathy through proximity, and to co-create with other choir members as the group collectively embodies these personal expressions for one another and for listeners.

Songwriting is not always easy. Challenging factors of songwriting include finding the courage and vulnerability to express what is in one's heart, developing the fortitude to experience the emotional content of the song or musical composition, listening to critical commentary about drafts of the song, and trusting others when sharing original ideas. An additional challenge may be reservations about the content and performances of original songs. This particular challenge arose when a member of the Oakdale Choir responded to a writing prompt that asked how the US national anthem might be rewritten from the perspective of people who are incarcerated.

Kenneth Bailey responded by writing the lyrics to a hopeful song, "Whispers from the Dawn." At the dress rehearsal for the performance, Kenneth read an introduction describing the prompt for the song and his response. After all the choir members had left the rehearsal, one of the prison activity staff approached me in the gym and told me that he was upset by Kenneth's introduction. This staff member had been deployed in Afghanistan and noted that many other people at Oakdale, both incarcerated individuals and staff, had been in the military as well. He said that from his perspective, it was disrespectful to question the lyrics in the US national anthem.

Is it not our role to think critically about commonly held practices? Why do people in custody not have this same opportunity to think critically and express their ideas? Nevertheless, with my position as volunteer and our need to continue to build positive relationships with all the prison staff and administrators, I asked Kenneth to revise his introduction.

The second time a prison official censored original material with the Oakdale Choir involved an original song, "Innocent Blood." Incarcerated African American songwriter Arnold Grice wrote the lyrics and music for it. Grice was reflecting on the Sandy Hook Elementary School shooting and asserting that it takes a village to support a community. The Deputy Warden refused to allow the performance of this song because he thought the title of the song referenced a gang. The Deputy Warden had not read the lyrics, nor listened to the song, nor spoken to Arnold. Arnold took these messages in stride and rewrote his song with a new title, "Love Lives On," which the choir performed successfully in a concert also themed "Love Lives On."

> In a world gone wrong, we pray that you'll stay strong
> And when the hurt hits home, just know that Love Lives On.
> And so we'll sing our song, with hopes that seeds are sown
> Trusting in God our cornerstone
> Knowing that Love Lives On. Remember Love Lives On.

In his song, Arnold acknowledges the deep hurt that people are experiencing, emphasizes how actions speak louder than words, and encourages us to realize that even amid grief, love lives on. The message was so popular among Oakdale Choir members that when the prison administration approved choir T-shirts, members voted for the message "Love Lives On" to be displayed the back of the shirts.

In this next story, songwriting provides insight into racial conflicts and misunderstandings among people who are incarcerated. One of Catherine Roma's many contributions has been that members of her Ohio prison choirs have created "new spirituals." With her strong background in a wide variety of musical styles, and her skills in building a "consensus model of decision making," she facilitates remarkable original compositions in funk, ballad, gospel, pop, and hip hop styles (Roma 2018, 23). These new spirituals provide a conduit for the singers to face their problems and comment on their life experiences. They invigorate the singers to solve personal issues while fostering a sense of belonging.[11]

Eddie Robertson, a member of Roma's choir, had written "Black Lives Matter" in 2015.[12] The title and theme of Eddie's original song were inspired by Alicia Garza, Patrisse Cullors, and Opal Tometi, who founded Black Lives Matter (BLM) in 2013 in response to the murder of seventeen-year-old Trayvon Martin, who was killed by George Zimmerman in Florida. Robertson was also reflecting on Tamir Rice, a twelve-year-old boy who was shot by a white police officer on November 22, 2014, while playing with a toy gun in a Cleveland park and who died the next day, and twenty-two-year old John Crawford III, who was killed by a police officer inside a Walmart in Beavercreek, Ohio, when Crawford was looking at a BB gun for sale. Eddie reported that the entire song took him only about an hour to compose:

1. Some of us don't believe in unity, we'd rather see hate be
     our reality.
   When will we see that love is the answer?
   We need to cure hate. It's more deadly than cancer.
   We're not afraid to speak up and reveal.
   This has united us. The movement is real.
   This can be solved, Let's get involved.
   Love is all around and we can make the difference.
   By looking at the evidence, we all can do better.

   CHORUS
   I'm telling you, Black Lives Matter.
   Inside the heart is where the change begins.
   Let's do it together.
   I'm telling you, Black Lives Matter.

2. I see brothers killin' brothers ev'ry night on the news.
   Well, it's a shame all they want is his shoes.
   Ev'rybody's talkin' but then nothin' gets done.

This is a call for unity.
We need ev'ryone.
Somehow we must do something,
I know there is a way,
Respectin' each other more and more ev'ry day.
Yes, you can change!
Don't stay the same!
Love is all around and it can make the difference!

FINAL CHORUS
You matter, I matter, I matter, forever, forever,
 Black Lives Matter.
She matters. He matters. He matters. They matter. I know that.
I'm tellin' you… Black Lives Matter. Black Lives Matter.
 Black Lives Matter.

The BLM movement is a political and ideological intervention that affirms Blacks' humanity, their contributions to society, and their resilience in a world in which they have been intentionally and systematically harmed. BLM shares with prominent US racial equality movements such as the civil rights movement a vision of economic equality and equal personhood. Eddie's song is a musical expression of that vision, yet the story of the first performance in the Madison Correctional Institution in Ohio by Roma's UBUNTU Choir illustrates how far the residents in this prison were from experiencing this ideal of equally valued personhood.

Eddie's original words "Black Lives Matter" were initially silenced and changed to the words "all lives matter" at the demand of Black prison authorities, who feared that the words "Black Lives Matter" might foment racial unrest in the prison. Given that several dignitaries were planning to attend, including state representatives and wardens, there was heightened concern about the potential negative outcome of those words. The prison authorities were employing an abundance of caution to avoid a situation in which the white residents of the facility would understand the message as "white lives do not matter." As a consequence, UBUNTU choir members sang the words "all lives matter" instead of "Black Lives Matter" throughout their concert performance of the song. After the performance, Eddie told Steve McQueen, a Community Voices producer for WYSO radio, that he was perplexed by the censorship of his song, and the ensuing conversation about the lyrics emboldened Eddie to educate both men in custody and staff about what it means to sing a song about the worth of Black lives, particularly inside a prison. Given the extreme racial disparities between whites and Blacks at all stages of the justice process in the US, Eddie's point is noteworthy: "If we can't sing about Black Lives Matter here in 2015, something is wrong with that picture. We need to examine what we're trying to talk about" (Robertson 2015).

Eddie himself and the choir he sang with were not allowed to perform the original lyrics expressing Eddie's position. Even so, Roma was able to record a CD with the UBUNTU Men's Chorus and the Ohio Voices for Justice, with Eddie soloing (Ubuntu Men's Chorus 2015). Her World House Choir created a YouTube video with the original lyrics to "Black Lives Matter." Both the audio recording and the video enabled Robertson's lyrical message to be heard beyond the prison walls, giving the general public insight into his message about prioritizing the worthiness and value of Black lives.[13]

Power dynamics are always at play in prisons and can negatively impact songwriting. These examples illustrate both the limitations the prison setting may impose on lyrical expression and the heightened need incarcerated individuals may have for such expressive outlets. In these cases, the prison authorities did not listen to the incarcerated individuals' thoughts or intentions; instead, their focus on security and control of expressive content curtailed the incarcerated individuals' opportunities to explain their song lyrics.

For a variety of reasons, it may be difficult to listen to other people's perspectives and the reasons why they take the positions they do. In a group choral setting, it is sometimes difficult to express vocally someone else's experiences in an original song. Different choir members have different life experiences and religious, cultural, and political views. One Oakdale choir member who had a strong religious identity composed a song that not all the choir members were comfortable singing, so those who were comfortable singing this song performed it in a smaller group. Through this experience the choir members discussed how to work through the tensions of singing about ideas one does not accept. Some members indicated that although it was difficult, the choir's roots in the concept of *ubuntu* provided the framework for realizing that although we have different individual beliefs, we can sing or listen to someone else's views in supportive solidarity. When choir members sing certain original songs, space is provided for people to become more open and aware of contrasting beliefs; this in turn provides a seed for learning to connect with others in more productive ways. Let's look at an example from 2005 in Kansas, where a rap composed in prison mixed with Gregorian chant was the basis of a protest.

Ten years before Robertson wrote "Black Lives Matter," the East Hill Singers performed an original composition titled "Rap of Redemption" that included a recording of Essex Simms's rap "I Wish I Never Hurt You" (Ranney 2005). In his rap, Simms apologizes for his crime of murder. Simms was unable to attend the performance in person because he was incarcerated in the maximum-security unit. The East Hill Singers chorus was in the minimum-security unit of the prison. The choir members with clean discipline records travelled outside the prison to join a group of men from the community for concerts. This performance piece started with a small chorus of twelve incarcerated and non-incarcerated men singing the Gregorian chant of the Greek text "Kyrie Eleison" (Lord have mercy, Christ have mercy, Lord have mercy), followed by an audio recording of Essex Simms performing his rap while the live voices hummed the melody "Of the Father's Love Begotten," based on the Latin poem "Corde natus." The stirring performance ended with the men singing the Gregorian chant of the Latin text "Agnus Dei" (Lamb of God you take away the sins of the world, have mercy on us. Grant us peace). It was premiered in Blessed Sacrament Catholic Church in Kansas City, Kansas.

According to journalist Jon Niccum, the Rev. Phillip Wolfe, leader of the church, was "incensed that rap music was going to be performed in a Catholic church" (Niccum 2006). After the congregants heard that the performance would include a song where rap was mixed with the traditional Gregorian chant they used in their worship services, fifty church members participated in a protest at the church the day of the concert. The protesters, all white, knelt in front of the church on cement steps and prayed the rosary. There was no discussion about the fact that Essex Simms was incarcerated and that his words were a contemporary expression of the ancient chants these congregants prayed each week. Voth expressed concern that the incarcerated singers thought the congregants were protesting them. News stories highlighted the protest, resulting in an overflow crowd for the second EHS concert the following week in Lawrence, Kansas, where additional audience members watched the performance live on a television screen in the church hall (Horsley 2006; Niccum 2006).

In this instance an original song, created in prison without dialogue about the meaning of the song and the choir's purpose, resulted in mistaken understandings and a missed opportunity to examine race relations. More than twelve years after this event, further creative applications of songwriting by people in custody are beginning to invite such conversations.

For example, artist/activist Fury Young combined songwriting with efforts to address systemic racism. In 2013 he began work on a concept album called *Die Jim Crow*, which featured predominantly formerly or currently incarcerated African Americans. Young was inspired by

Occupy Wall Street and provoked after reading Michelle Alexander's book, *The New Jim Crow*, which argues the US prison system has legalized discrimination and created a new caste system by locking up millions of African Americans, relegating them to second-class status (Alexander 2010). "Die Jim Crow," Young notes, basically signifies "death to the idea of the 'Other'"—that is, death to stereotypes. After recording more than fifty musicians in five different prisons between 2015 and 2019, Young expanded the idea into a record label whose mission is to provide formerly and currently incarcerated musicians with a high-quality platform for society to listen to their voices.[14] These individuals include Albert Woodfox, who served forty-three years in solitary confinement in the Louisiana State Penitentiary in Angola, and four rappers in youth facilities in Mississippi (Kaplan 2020). Die Jim Crow Records has released more than thirty-five original songs. Through crowd sourcing, the DJC record label has raised money to provide protective equipment for people in custody during the Covid-19 pandemic.

August Tarrier created a similar not-for-profit called Songs in the Key of Free.[15] It first collaborated with musicians incarcerated in State Correctional Institution – Graterford in Pennsylvania, who wrote and recorded a concept album, *Rise*, addressing mass incarceration. It then added voices of non-incarcerated musicians into the recording. Songs in the Key of Free aims to convey the dignity and humanity of people who have been justice-involved. Its podcast, Prison Prophets, launched in 2019.[16] Its efforts resonate with abolitionist thinking:

> Songs in the Key of Free addresses the wounds inflicted by the carceral state. Our aim is to dismantle the boundaries it imposes, the silence it imposes, to counter its vast power—one human at a time. One body, one voice, joined with other bodies and other voices in a chorus to take back our bodies, our voices, and our stories.[17]

Yet another example of recorded voices of musicians in custody aiming to change social narratives involves a sculpture exhibition inside the former Eastern State Penitentiary in Philadelphia. ESP was the world's first "penitentiary" and was designed for people in custody to be in solitude for penance and punishment. The building now holds a museum. Jess Perlitz, an art professor at Lewis and Clark College in Oregon, asked people in custody which one song they would sing for people to hear outside of prisons. She collected audio recordings, including some original songs from people incarcerated throughout the country. When people enter her exhibit "Chorus," they enter a narrow, rectangular, enclosed space with one small rectangular window in the ceiling. Motion detectors set off a series of audio recordings of their voices singing.[18] They first hear one voice singing, then another voice starts, and this continues until a cacophony of voices are layered onto one another. Perlitz says that according to the feedback she's received, participants who attend the exhibit can feel the performers' vulnerability, bravery, and earnestness, different from what is typically represented in newspapers and films (Jess Perlitz, pers. comm. to Mary Cohen, January 11, 2021).

Most recently, Terri Lynne Carrington, a three-time Grammy winner as well as a recipient of the National Endowment for the Arts Jazz Masters Award, curated and directed "Music for Abolition," a collection of fifteen original songs and videos that express grief, exhaustion, rage, and resolution, resonating with calls of freedom, and sounding a shared struggle for abolition.[19] From a Black feminist foundation, these original songs have been co-created through a collective process that parallels the process for abolishing the prison industrial complex. Mariame Kaba, cited in our introductory chapter, argues for employing collective responsibility and for being in purposeful relation to one another in order to move toward abolishing harmful carceral logics (Kaba 2021, 4).

Songwriting and group music-making can serve as examples of the new collective structures that Kaba calls for. Such collaborations are an important step toward growing the conversation about abolitionist thinking, as the musical expressions provide innovative and creative contributions to the discourse. More regular opportunities to build relationships between people who are in custody and people from the community are necessary to build motivation for imagining healing forms of justice.

Roma's musical facilitation of Black musical styles has provided musical outlets for incarcerated individuals to express themselves through original songs and new spirituals. One of the original songs, "Begin to Love," by Eddie Robertson, who has sung with Roma for years and was spared from his initial death sentence by a judge, includes the words "It only matters that people around the world begin to love." Robertson's message is vital to the process of building caring communities.

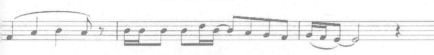

CHAPTER 6

"SO MUCH MORE"

Pedagogies That Support Human Dignity and Social Responsibility for Musical Communities Working toward Abolition of the Prison Industrial Complex

Although there is literature that examines pedagogy and pedagogical frameworks employed within prisons, there has been, as far as we know, little discussion of music-making and musical community formation in prisons from a pedagogical perspective. Throughout this book we have focused on several individual instrumental, vocal, and songwriting programs within spaces of incarceration across the US. Now we consider how people can apply the theoretical frameworks, individual pedagogies, and music activities inspired by the musical programs explored in prior chapters. In the process, we consider how these applications align with practices that work to dismantle the prison industrial complex.

As Rebecca Ginsburg has argued, any college-in-prison program that is poorly designed or ineffectively implemented is likely to do more harm than good. She contends that "when instructors who are headed behind the wall are not aware of the challenges and risks of prison teaching, they are more likely to take on the values and imperatives of the carceral state and their classrooms and programs are likely to become yet another repressive force in incarcerated individuals' lives" (Ginsburg 2019, 1).[1] Music educators inside and outside prisons face similar challenges if they have not critically examined their pedagogies, the musical styles they offer their students, or the cultural practices and lifestyles of their learners.

Eric Shieh, a music educator and former facilitator of music programs in a Michigan prison, models a critically reflective stance about his teaching in prisons (Shieh 2010). He responded to this question: What are the most important things people need to know related to any aspect of facilitating musical learning in a prison?

> That I am implicated in the system of mass incarceration in the U.S., and that my work must be engaged in solidarity with the incarcerated, their families, and advocates for the reform of our justice system....We are engaged mutually in finding out what music will mean to us, my role must at some level be one of a facilitator of musical engagements, of emergent knowledges. (Eric Shieh, response to questionnaire, October 23, 2016)

A music educator in a prison provides resources and experiences for learners to explore, affirm, and celebrate their humanity through musical expressions, even while surrounded by systems of control and harm that we, along with many other thinkers, researchers, and activists, argue need to be disrupted, overhauled, and transformed at the local, state, and national levels. Simultaneously developing music-making activities inside prisons, creating and furthering public awareness, and inspiring innovative changes requires, at a minimum, relationship-building, listening, and fostering an awareness of the power dynamics that occur within individual prisons, along with a solid theoretical framework based on culturally sustaining pedagogies applied to music-making.

Power dynamics are embedded throughout criminal legal systems—in the establishment of laws, in policing, during trials and sentencing, within correctional facilities, and in community supervision. As we have seen in a number of prison programs discussed in earlier chapters, correctional staff's interactions with people in custody fall on a continuum from supportive to dehumanizing. We saw how relationships among people who are incarcerated range from encouraging and supportive to problematic and outright harmful. And, most importantly, we saw the need for relationship-building with administrators and among participants in order to simply establish these programs, let alone help them flourish across changes in prison leadership, membership in musical ensembles, state or national policies and approaches, and musical leadership.

Power dynamics occur in all aspects of incarceration. In many ways, the very constructs by which music-making courses are designed constitute a method of control. In music education contexts, structuring rehearsals and planning how to learn new pieces are themselves acts of control. And where the physical space, the dress code, and the surveillance of correctional officers all serve as constant reminders of that control for incarcerated students, it is all the more important for leaders of music programs to examine the control that their syllabus and teaching plans exhibit, and adopt student-centred and culturally relevant and sustaining pedagogies.

A syllabus is in itself not a locus of control; rather, it is the conduit through which control is exerted. A facilitator of learning sets expectations, including course content, assignments for completion, due dates for completion, and grading. This last element, grading, can be the one that leads to the most harm if not carefully considered, but conversely, it can allow for individual growth for an incarcerated student. Though it can generate stress and confusion for incarcerated students, grading can also serve as a form of validation. That validation is closely associated with identity-building and self-worth, both of which, as we have seen, are suppressed within incarcerated environments.

With all this in mind, during a music appreciation class I (Stuart Duncan) taught in 2010 at Auburn Correctional Facility (ACF), a maximum-security prison in New York state, I tried a different form of assessment that foregrounded the role of the incarcerated student and their own understanding of their learning (Duncan 2013). The course was a part of a larger collection of courses offered through the Cornell Prison Education Program. This program, which is still active, aids incarcerated students in completing an associate degree. It includes faculty, staff, and graduate and undergraduate teaching assistants from Cornell University and Cayuga Community College.

Many of the experiences I have had while teaching bear similarities to the journeys we have shared with other musical leaders in this book. However, there is one unique element in this program that adds to the "how" regarding our first point, about developing one's sense of self. In ACF, grades do not hold quite the same level of urgency, yet they are still seen by many of the incarcerated students as a means of control very similar to other modes of control that make up so much of their incarceration experience. I wanted to flip this power dynamic on its head by empowering students rather than coercing and enforcing certain types of learning through grade shaming.

Instead of the traditional grading, I established one-to-one contracts with each student after the first few weeks, highlighting their current achievements, identifying potential growth areas, and exploring what goals they might want to set. I met each student individually and asked them to reflect on whether my assessment of their achievements matched their own. These growth areas were always framed with students' interests in mind. The two parties negotiated, altered, confirmed, and agreed to the contracts. At the end of the semester, we met individually again, and I asked the students to assess themselves based on this contract. I showed them the grade I had tentatively assigned, and then we again negotiated and resolved any concerns. What was fascinating to me was that most students assigned the same grade that I had or had given themselves one half-step lower (a B– instead of a B, for example). Only one student had graded himself significantly higher and did not care for the grading system.

On reflection, this process of contract grading empowered the students; it gave them voice and an occasion to consider both their own and someone else's views. They experienced how negotiation, rather than conflict, could play a role in shaping an end result. They also took responsibility for their own learning: this was for them, not me, to judge. This flipping of the power dynamic shifted the question from "Have you completed what the course set out to achieve" to "How do you feel about the goals you have set yourself and where you are at in meeting them?" Upon finishing the semester, one student said to me, "This is the first time I've felt like a human being in many years." He explained that the contract grading was one of the elements that had helped him change how he viewed his own conversations with others and realize that conflict could be mitigated through negotiation, self-reflection, and understanding someone else's point of view.[2] I have never forgotten that experience, and while the focus of this book has been on musicking as a change agent for our students and society, as instructors, we too can be changed. We also learn from these experiences, hopefully as much as our students do.

This teaching and learning process, where negotiation and dialogue are a core part of class experience, can differ from the pedagogies of many performance-based musical ensembles. Traditionally, group music-making includes a musical leader, commonly called a "director." This leader conveys control of an ensemble through gesture, language, arrangement of musicians, content, and instruction. Musical leaders also often make choices about musical styles and pedagogical approaches.

Some choices, however inadvertently, can result in students feeling alienated, belittled, or shamed. Yet other choices can create a sense of collaboration, equality, affirmation, and empowerment.

In choirs, participants work together toward common goals such as group expression of lyrics arranged melodically, rhythmically, and in a style or idiom structure, traditionally in preparation for a performance. Accordingly, the leader's philosophy, purpose, instructional choices, and personality influence the level of collaboration and social growth among members. When choir leaders encourage members to welcome new members into the learning space and when all students build a sense of hospitality (Higgins 2012), mutually caring relationships are created, allowing the choir to meet its musical, expressive, and social goals more effectively and more satisfactorily.

In my (Cohen's) theory of interactional choral singing pedagogy, I offer that if musical leaders facilitate interactions effectively, opportunities unfold that can result in measurable personal and social growth (Cohen 2007a, 292–96). Music educators can build their skills for effective interactions by studying culturally responsive pedagogies as applied to music ensembles (Shaw 2020). Researchers have tested the theory of interactional choral singing pedagogy and found that through choral singing, outside leaders, participants, and audience members all experience personal as well as social growth. For example, volunteers and audience members who come inside a prison to sing with people who are incarcerated or to participate in a musical performance increase their awareness of people in prison (Cohen 2012a; Messerschmidt 2017). Members of the public who have not previously thought about incarcerated individuals have an experience that humanizes people behind bars. Some members of the public will have been survivors of crimes, and their perceptions are important to consider when studying pedagogies for music-making in prisons.

In the fall of 2018, I (Cohen) hosted a listening panel in the Voxman Music Building on the University of Iowa campus with survivors of violent crime, outside Oakdale Choir members, and Warden Jim McKinney to hear their perspectives on music education in prisons. We learned how the perpetrator and the survivors hold an unusual connection through their shared experience with the crime. Many survivors commented how immediately after the crime, they were furious with the perpetrator. It took them time to find a space of forgiveness. One generative outcome of our session was the idea of inviting a victim of a crime to come to a choir rehearsal and discuss their experiences. In November, a survivor of child sexual abuse talked with the choir about his experiences. It was optional for members to attend, and some chose not to come. Those inside singers who did come were extremely appreciative that a man had chosen to share his stories of trauma and healing. They expressed admiration for his perseverance through many years of successes and challenges and for his willingness to be so vulnerable while at the same time showing a very real yet gentle strength. Such dialogues highlight the complex and often traumatic personal histories of many individuals. These conversations also speak to the need for effective behavioural health services both in the community and while incarcerated.

Survivors of violent crimes often express painful feelings, and the process for them to work through their feelings can be long and difficult. Researchers have contended that crime survivors' interests align with efforts to decarcerate through addressing underlying drivers of crime and balancing community needs, defendants' rights and interests, and rights (Krinsky and Komar 2021). Survivors of crime may not be interested in attending musical performances or participating in a prison program; even so, music educators teaching in prisons need to consider crime survivors' views and work to apply innovative approaches to creating spaces for listening to their stories and feelings. For example, through the Iowa Department of Corrections' Office of Victim and Restorative Justice Programs, I received a poem written by a crime survivor, Elma Ingamells. Ingamells allowed the Oakdale Songwriting Workshop participants to create lyrics based on her poem, "Inside a Mother's Heart," and set it to music. She attended the informal performance inside the prison testing room, where a group of twelve incarcerated men sang the song. Ingamells described to me how that experience had helped "heal her heart." She noted that when she heard the songwriters perform a song based on her poem, it was one of several factors that helped her realize that people are more than the worst thing they have done and that she is more than a victim. No one is completely defined by a single behaviour; the musical collaboration validated her worth and created an awareness of the perpetrators' worth. Sometimes family members of people in custody are the survivors of crimes, so holding no assumptions about anyone's perceptions or experiences is a vital aspect of developing an effective pedagogy for incarcerated students.

For community members with little or no personal experience with people in custody, musical performances introduce them to some of the human experiences of incarcerated populations and allow them to empathize with the performers. The interactions at these events can lead community members to reflect on their experiences and may challenge their preconceptions about incarcerated people. For community members who take an active role in challenging the PIC, musical performances and learning exchanges designed to combine musical performance with dialogue offer spaces for information sharing, listening, and conversation.

Not everything about musical performance in this context is free from challenges. Amanda Weber, founder and leader of the Voices of Hope Women's Prison Choir in Minnesota, cautions that people could potentially leave a concert or a rehearsal inside a prison overconfident, believing that they know the ins and outs of prisons. If they think they are experts on this highly complex topic, they may contribute to further misconceptions in their conversations with others who have little or no awareness of prisons. Moreover, she warns that if outside volunteers' internal change does not result in external actions, the people who primarily benefit will be the majority status group and there will be no efforts to dismantle the PIC (Weber 2018, 154–56). In her recognition of racial injustice in imprisonment in the US, Weber suggests that members of society, especially those participating in music-making in prisons, must "reflect on our own identity formation and our commitment to one another" (169) rather than feeling like they are "called to help." Weber calls on us to recognize how our beliefs, our biases, and our lack of listening to and understanding the complex stories of people impacted by prisons can inadvertently perpetuate harmful systems. In addition to this, we need to commit to living in a way that acknowledges our common humanity and practise empathy, forgiveness, and compassion for ourselves and others.

Musical leaders in prisons require a variety of pedagogical tools to create mutually respectful relationships with and among all involved; they must also incorporate a culturally relevant and sustaining pedagogical framework. Other theoretical approaches such as restorative justice and peacebuilding practices emphasize a collaborative "with" approach in order to develop mutual trust, rather than a "sage on the stage" mentality (Cohen and Duncan 2015). Karin Hendricks illustrates how participants' authentic voices and stories can be expressed more easily when healthy relationships between instructor and students have been established (Hendriks 2018). According to Hendricks, building trust has two central components: let the learners govern themselves; and support the learners to guide one another.

Given that incarcerated individuals have little autonomy, promoting rather than suppressing participant input can help group members feel empowered. However, some musical participants may find such autonomy uncomfortable in an ensemble setting, and others may not wish to provide input, so understanding the individual needs of each ensemble member, and guiding them toward developing their agency, is paramount. A musical leader must allow for a wide variety of levels of participation in the prison-based ensemble, affirming participants' potential and inviting opportunities for shared leadership. It is necessary to critically consider which types of arts-based approaches support human dignity and social responsibility, and how to facilitate those approaches in a manner that builds a sense of personal and communal respect.

In acknowledgement of potentially harmful power dynamics in a prison-based music education program, André de Quadros and his colleagues Emily Howe, Jamie Hillman, and Trey Pratt created an arts-based experiential learning process that is collaborative, anti-authoritarian, mutually respectful, egalitarian, and inclusive—one that also fosters tenderness and creates space for participants to be vulnerable (de Quadros 2015; 2016, 188–89). Called "Empowering Song," their approach focuses on "healing, consolation, love, personal expression, and community mobilization" (Howe et al. 2020, 114). They designed and led a series of workshops at MCI for men in Norfolk and MCI for women in Framingham through improvised storytelling, poetry, drama, visual arts, bodywork, song creation, theatre, and dance (de Quadros and Amrein forthcoming). In the Empowering Song approach in these two Massachusetts Correctional Institutions, there were no public performances. Rather, the emphasis was on communal interaction. Around twenty people met weekly for three hours per session. For the men's program, they used themes based on songs such as the phrase "And neither have I wings to fly" from the song "O Waly" or "I once was lost but now am found" from "Amazing Grace." Other themes were developed from phrases such as the traditional Persian Sufi saying, "This too shall pass" (de Quadros 2018, 271–72).

Empowering Song student Derrick Washington described his first class "as a brief transfer from a world of hell to a world of relief" (Washington 2020, 289). Derrick assumed that the Boston University music class would take a teacher-centred approach focusing on classical composers and reading musical scores. However, Empowering Song includes co-created content and is based on concepts in Augusto Boal's *Theatre of the Oppressed* (1985) and *The Aesthetics of the Oppressed*

(2006). Theatre of the Oppressed is an interactive, embodied, playful experience in which participants explore alternative responses to oppressive situations. Boal wrote, "I have sincere respect for those artists who dedicate their lives exclusively to their art—it is their right or their condition—but I prefer those who dedicate their art to life" (Boal 1985, 107). De Quadros has dedicated his art and pedagogical approach to supporting the learners' lives through critical examinations of the oppressed and the oppressor and affirming the individual humanity of each participant. When Derrick walked into the classroom where the rows of desks, chairs, and tables had been pushed against the walls, de Quadros welcomed him with "a really kind handshake greeting in which the energy he conveyed was really comforting as if I had been a beloved family member of a longtime friend." Derrick felt a sense of "temporarily restored dignity and a sense of humanity" (Washington 2020, 290). He noted that this first class changed his perception of music as well as how he interacted with people. A transformation, he noted, that he can apply the rest of his life (292).

Empowering Song student Ismael "Q" Garcia-Vega's mother was addicted to heroin. When Ismael was nine, she gave him to one of her dealers and he was molested while his mom got high. He almost lost his life to suicide at age ten. By age fourteen he had been stabbed, shot at, and run over by a truck, finally reaching a breaking point where he became the predator in order to stop being the victim; he became a founding member of a gang in his city. Between time in a juvenile detention centre and adult facilities, he had served over eighteen years in custody before participating in Empowering Song (Garcia-Vega 2020, 166).

Ismael described how at his first Empowering Song class he sat across the circle from a rival gang member who had recently attacked one of his gang members. A warm-up for a session involved the participants standing in a circle holding hands, singing, and moving together. They stretched, breathed mindfully, and centred. They improvised original songs (de Quadros 2016, 188–89). Holding hands in a men's prison?

De Quadros did not tell them in advance they were going to hold hands, rather as he spoke about something else, he easily held the hands of the two people next to him, and everyone in the circle followed his lead. Ismael noted that this experience of holding hands and seeing the others join in the circle was transformational.

For Ismael, before this experience, he had associated the role of hands in human contact with the physical abuse he had received at his father's hands. The following week, de Quadros asked his class how holding hands felt. They indicated that holding hands made them feel uncomfortable. For some, it likely made them confront, physically and emotionally, their own frames of reference with regard to their perceptions of manhood and masculinity. De Quadros had taken a risk by involving incarcerated students in a vulnerable activity early in their group learning experiences, yet doing so set the stage for a classroom environment that challenged preconceptions. This approach seemed to work in this context, but there was a sense of power at play with de Quadros as an outside professor leading the men to hold hands, and it is difficult to understand how each participant experienced it. The men described their sense of vulnerability, and de Quadros acknowledged and affirmed how vulnerability in artmaking was vital and critical to the work.

Wayland "X" Coleman had served twenty-two years in Massachusetts prisons before participating in the Empowering Song class. He explained how all the activities affected different people in different ways. Interactions with teachers and guests from outside the prison altered his previous view that people did not care about them. He had to relinquish his anger with the world (Coleman 2020, 100–101). For Wayland, the changes were not behavioural. He noted, "I was given a new way to look at where I stood in relation to the world, to society, and to people individually" (99). Wayland felt a deep sense of healing, rehumanizing activism, and this change stood in contrast to the oppression, repression, and institutionalization he had long been used to feeling. He noted that the prison administration and staff had begun to scrutinize the Empowering Song class more than any of the other courses offered through Boston University's Prison Education Program. The prison staff restricted what supplies the professors could bring in and what the students could turn in for assignments (102). According to Wayland, "the system wanted control over anything that could cause us to understand our human value" (102).

An Empowering Song activity that promotes deep human dignity and social responsibility is where one person comes to the centre of a circle of singers and closes their eyes. The people in the circle then sing that person's name. De Quadros has noted that this activity has been life-changing every time he leads it (de Quadros 2018, 270). The power of receiving one's name as a vocal symphony from an entire community requires vulnerability and builds dignity, group caring, and a sense of shared responsibility through co-creation.

One of the most important outcomes that can arise from programs like de Quadros's Empowering Song is that it helps incarcerated students gain important skills for re-entry into society. Shadd Maruna, a criminology professor at Queen's University Belfast, contends that the lack of rituals supporting returning citizens may explain some of the difficulties of re-entry. The term "ritual" is important here; it refers to solidarity and social cohesion enacted through community bonding for a common cause. Such "rites of passage" shape human lives, and when successful they create feelings of belonging and acceptance. In some groups such as fraternities or youth gangs, ritualistic behaviours such as hazing and vandalism are harmful, yet they still serve a purpose of communal bonding (Maruna 2011, 7–10). Arrests, jail time or bail, trials, and incarceration are full of rituals, but the processes of re-entry are not. Indeed, criminal punishments end inadequately, and in many cases they do not end at all (Maruna 2011, 5).[3] Maruna suggests that through a deeper understanding of roles and rituals in human life,[4] these ideas can be applied to supporting returning individuals. He posits that reintegration rituals have four key aspects: they are symbolic and emotive, they repeat as necessary, they involve community, and they focus on challenge and achievement instead of risk of reoffending (3–28). Music-making in prisons touches on and engenders an experience of each of these four (Cohen 2019b).

First, musical creating and performing is highly symbolic and emotive. Effectively facilitated songwriting is a personally expressive activity that provides a means for people in custody to connect with one another, build friendships, and express difficult and deeply felt emotions (Wilson 2013). A songwriting workshop in a men's prison led to the development of personal identity, internal locus of control, intensive involvement with the task at hand, and a sense of fulfillment (Cohen and Wilson 2017, 543–51).

Second, music-making in prisons involves several ritualistic and repeated aspects. Choral rehearsals regularly begin with physical and vocal warm-ups and involve repetition of musical selections as the group learns arrangements and prepares singers for a performance, and many times they end with a closing song. Year after year, musical ensembles tend to repeat a schedule of preparation, performance, and recognition of the performance, and this offers a sense of engaging in seasonal rituals. Individual musical study and practice also include repetition and rituals.

Third, musical programs in prisons involve community in multiple ways. The programs may include people from outside the prison as part of the performing musical ensemble. Also, music-making creates community within the prison and builds relationships among participants (Douglas 2019). When people from the community come into a prison to attend performances, a direct connection is created between inside the prison and the outside community. When communities outside prison perform original songs by incarcerated songwriters or when radio shows or podcasts broadcast those original songs, the public can listen to incarcerated voices.

Fourth and finally, musical creation and performance focuses on challenge and achievement, thus creating a space for strength-based growth. Healthy risk-taking is part of the processes of songwriting, musical learning, and performing, and with supportive pedagogical and social environments, musicians inside and outside prisons can experience a sense of achievement within the risk-taking aspects of musical activities. Additionally, growth through music-making can carve out spaces to develop new relationships and strengthen current relationships. This seeds social cohesion.

In a musical group inside a prison, social cohesion can ebb, flow, and evolve. One way to develop a new musical community is by creating and practising simple rituals within rehearsals, such as singing anchoring songs at the beginning and end of practices and concerts. Such practices and other ritual aspects of music-making can become part of reintegration rituals.

With respect to the performative aspects of music education programs in prisons, these experiences provide opportunities for personal empowerment and family connections as well as positive social change. One Voices of Hope participant exclaimed after a performance, "I'm in treatment, and I have *never* felt a high like that!" (Weber 2018, 105). This type of success motivates further participation in the musical ensemble and inspires participation in other educational and musical experiences during and after release from prison. As Elvera Voth repeatedly asked, can you imagine how it feels to receive a standing ovation, when your entire life you have been called worthless?

An invitation for audience members to share their reflections with the director and singers encourages another type of social interaction. At the end of concerts, feedback sessions and conversations between audience members and performers provide opportunities to debrief and reflect on their musical experiences. A receiving line and fellowship, if possible, through sharing food and drink after performances, creates connections between audience members and performers. These social interactions have repeatedly allowed incarcerated singers to feel worthy, accepted, and affirmed. Building meaningful relationships with family, political leaders, legal professionals, and grassroots organizers can create a space for being in relation with one another. This is a necessary incremental step toward the broader goals of developing abolitionist thinking, imagining healing justice, and dismantling the PIC.

Creating space for meaningful social interactions can involve many paths. It is important for leaders to consider and implement purposeful pedagogical practices that are appropriate for their context, as well as consider the larger community that surrounds and supports the people involved, all the while broadly aware of the need to build responsivity and to overhaul systems rooted in harm and violence. In prisons, this larger community includes the survivors of crimes, the families of those survivors, the families of the incarcerated musicians, and employees of the prison and their families.

For arts instructors to be agents of change, they must realize how complex, individualized, and difficult life can be for people in prison. Music educator Eric Shieh described times when he felt completely, utterly ineffective—for example, when a participant self-constrained on the floor, face-down, to try to control his anger. Many incarcerated individuals have regularly been told they are worthless, both directly and indirectly through complicated legal processes and other interactions. If the musical community is an ensemble preparing for a performance, the teacher-conductor needs to figure out ethical and effective ways to communicate constructive feedback. Instructions for vocal or instrumental techniques, improving vocal projection and tone, and refining musicality need to be communicated as productively as possible. When the instructor needs to say something to a specific individual, it is best to take an affirming approach before or after rehearsal—perhaps with humour and a clear understanding that the individual's participation is appreciated and that their worth is valued.

A wound festers if conditions do not allow for healing. The ideology of punishment as a solution for social, economic, and political problems is illogical; it also limits society's ability to explore new possibilities for addressing root issues. Historically, prisons were places where people accused of crimes were held until they were whipped, used as slaves, or killed.[5] In the nineteenth century, punishment took the form of separating people from society in the mistaken belief that this would deter people from committing crimes. There is no conclusive evidence that prisons reduce criminal behaviour; indeed, researchers report that imprisonment has a criminogenic effect (Cook and Haynes 2021). Furthermore, victimization while in custody leads to offending and substance abuse, adding to the turmoil in both their lives and their communities. Arts and music education programming, however, leads to more caring and resilient neighbours. Now, many entities are working toward positive transformative changes, and Maruna (2017) has suggested a new social movement is growing where formerly incarcerated individuals, researchers, and activists are collaborating and creating supportive communities. Music-making in prisons can be a key part of this process.

Throughout this book we have illustrated how music education can be a means for people in custody to achieve personal and social growth. It can also create opportunities to achieve social awareness of the problems of the prison industrial complex. We have provided case studies of past and contemporary musical communities that have demonstrated these outcomes for participants and listeners. Meaningful social cohesion and social transformation to disrupt the systemically harmful aspects of prisons will require personal and social changes both inside and outside prison walls.

We conclude with the lyrics to an original song that encapsulates the idea that building relationships, in order to create collective care and social responsibility, starts by freeing one's authentic voice. Oakdale Choir member Arnold Grice introduced his original song "So Much More" with a message of hope for the audience: "We all face some trials and tribulations in this life, I just want to let you know to be encouraged. It doesn't matter whether you are in prison or whether you're free. Keep your head up."

His lyrics begin by uncovering the complex identities of people in custody:

> I am So Much More … than this number on my ID
> I am So Much More … than your excuse not to like me
> I am So Much More … than this charge to my conviction
> I am So Much More … than all your negative predictions
> I am So Much More … than the title of offender
> I am So Much More … than last place on your agenda
> I am So Much More … than just a neighborhood felon
> I am So Much More … than just a victim of the system … [6]

The words we use infuse or confuse the actions we choose. Negative labels reinforce stereotypes and "reduce" the individual. These labels limit our ability to connect with one another. Terms such as *offender, felon, prisoner, inmate,* and *victim* contribute to these misunderstandings. Music-making in prisons provides opportunities for "delabelling." Thomas Meisenhelder (1982, 137–53), a sociologist at California State University, San Bernardino, describes it as "social verification of the individual's reform." Delabelling processes are vital for people who have been incarcerated so that they can reintegrate effectively into society; perhaps just as important, they are vital for people outside of prisons so that they can be open to the deeper historical and social stories of individuals impacted by imprisonment.

Over the course of this book, we have foregrounded the power that music-making can wield both inside and outside prison walls for those who are incarcerated, their families and friends, and the community at large. This power relies on building human relationships. Starting with the discussion on the rise of mass incarceration in the US and of the horrifying rise of the PIC, we have outlined how the carceral state strips individuals of their own self-esteem and creates systems that prevent the building of relationships. Prior to the excessive caging of human bodies, music-making was a more regular practice in prisons. Evidence indicates that these experiences created opportunities for personal and social growth for people in custody. Today's harsh punitive approaches and extreme sentences are such that people in society *must* somehow change their perceptions and stop relying on prisons as a safety mechanism. We have shown that instrumental and vocal music programs, and other forms of musical instruction, can be impactful in this regard. However, this comes with an important caveat: music is not a panacea, nor is it immune from harmful outcomes. More research is needed to examine how concepts such as restorative and transformative practices, strength-based and culturally relevant and sustaining pedagogies, and desistance and reintegration rituals can be safely and effectively utilized not just in musical experiences but in other arts programming and educational approaches in prisons.

The musical experiences led by Duncan, de Quadros, Cohen, and Weber that we have discussed in this closing chapter offer different entry points and avenues for exploration for applying these pedagogies. Much more work must be done to begin healing the harms of mass incarceration and dismantling carceral logics that have made the US the world leader in warehousing humans. Music-making is just a small pebble in a pond, but with the right people and pedagogies, the ripples that emanate may start to move the needle toward addressing those harms. Music-making is not just about the individual incarcerated students; it is also about how music can bring incarcerated people together to share positive and affirming experiences for those outside of prison walls, thereby creating an enhanced awareness of the complexities of prisons and transforming cultures of revenge into communities of caring and a more deeply felt social responsibility.

A NOTE ON THE COVER

A few words about my painting, "Jazz Band."

The year spent at C-Yard, Solidad State Prison, was memorable for me, in a time of my life I'd sooner forget, for it was there I was introduced to Jack Bowers and the program he directed, Arts in Corrections. AIC provided art and music lessons, materials, and instruments to creative residents.

Twice a week, or as often as possible, I'd walk the long, dreary corridor to the AIC lab, where jazz music could often be heard emanating through its doors as I approached. Jack and his band of resident players would be there jamming out as I found my way to my corner, where I'd paint canvases and murals with the generous art materials at hand. What a terrific environment! There I was, painting away to the sounds of live jazz!

One day, I turned my canvas toward the band and "recorded" what I saw as the band played on. That moment lives on in the painting, "Jazz Band." I think the vibrant colours capture the joyful vibe of the musicians.

Jack bought that painting from me when he saw it, which honoured me. It made me feel human, that he thought so much of my work.

I think Jack and the AIC program helped a lot of the residents of that cold place feel more human.

—Jason Chengrian

The musical excerpt on the front cover is from an original song, "Remember: Be Love," by Michael Blackwell, Sr. and Rebecca Swanson. The lyrics that go with this portion of the melody are: "Every wrong is the reason to forgive." The Oakdale Choir performance recording is on the choir's website, at *https://oakdalechoir.lib.uiowa.edu/2019/12/12/ remember-be-love*.

ACKNOWLEDGEMENTS

STUART P. DUNCAN

This project has been a labour of love, stretching for over a decade. During that time, much of my life has changed, and with each new stage my relationship with the research has gained new insights and perspectives. Since first talking with Mary in 2010, I completed doctorates at Cornell and Yale, got married, had a child, changed career trajectory, and, like all of us, navigated a pandemic. But through all these changes it has been an absolute delight to work with Mary, and to challenge each other in the ways we think about music, education, pedagogy, incarceration, and larger societal issues. And of course, I would not have had the energy needed for this book without the support of the love of my life, Jen (and, of course, our two dogs, Benson and Clover).

GRATITUDE FOR COMMUNITIES OF CARE BY MARY L. COHEN

As I reflect upon the multitude of people and experiences that have played a role in developing this book, it is so clear to me that I am surrounded and grounded with communities of care. How awesome to be aware of and to acknowledge all these meaningful, insightful, and special influences upon my life and this book. My co-author Stuart Paul Duncan has been a rock and a brilliant thinker, critical and creative, supportive and resilient. Through over ten years building this project together, we've seen each other through many life transitions, including the birth of his son; the deaths of my sister Judy, brother Joe, and my dad; Stuart's completion of his PhD in music theory at Yale; my promotion to associate professor with tenure at the University of Iowa; my ten years as area head of the music education department; and over eleven years of my founding and facilitating the Oakdale Prison Community Choir and songwriting workshop. We've supported one another, challenged one another's writing, discussed related difficult topics, and completed this book.

Varied communities of care have supported me and influenced my thinking and work on this book. I express my deepest gratitude to these individuals and groups, both named and unnamed, and attempt to describe them in eight different yet related categories.

Family. My dear, supportive, loving, and caring husband, Matt: thank you, lovely, for all your consistent support, encouragement, playful energy, calming presence, and love. My gratitude flows deeply for you. My inspirational departed sister, Judy: you know how you have influenced me in all the things I enjoy in life—music, well-being, scholarly explorations. Thank you for your guidance. I am so grateful for my parents, Paul and Louise Shinogle, who provided me with necessities and privileges—piano lessons, my undergraduate education, encouragement through health challenges, and so many prayers. Thank you to my siblings Jane, Joe, Bob, and Linda; my niece Laurel, nephews Ralph, Charlie, Andy, and Ben; my in-laws Jackie, Miles, Ruth, John, Micah, and Noah. Huge gratitude to my spiritual wellness friends, Sandy Kemp, Mary Thompson, Maria Peth, and Jennifer Shoals. Thank you to Bob Roth for leading the twice-daily Transcendental Meditations that began in March 2020. Thank you to Prairiewoods Franciscan Spirituality Center and the staff who have been a source of renewal through difficult experiences as well as advocates for the Oakdale Choir.

Readers. Deepest gratitude to everyone who has read and provided comments on drafts of our manuscript. Mary Trachsel, your critical commentary, and edits have been beyond remarkable. Thank you for your thoughtful, detailed, and productive insights. Kirstin Anderson, thank you for reading early drafts and important insistence to use people-centred language. Thank you to all the incarcerated readers who gave us important points and considerations we would not have thought of on our own. Thanks also to Thom Gehring and Carolyn Eggleston for your insights regarding correctional education. Thank you to Andy Douglas, Barbara Eckstein, Nancy Halder, Amanda McLearn-Montz, and Dorothy Whiston. Thank you to the blind reviewers facilitated by Wilfrid Laurier University Press. We so appreciate your time, energy, and commentary on our book.

Kansas. Elvera Voth: you are a true rock star. Thank you for your creative inspiration to start the East Hill Singers, build the not-for-profit organization Arts in Prison, Inc., bring together community musicians with the Lansing Correctional Facility singers, and allow me to learn from you and everyone in your organization. My work as a special projects coordinator during graduate school at the University of Kansas provided a vital introduction to the role of arts in prisons and sparked my interest in exploring this topic in more depth. Thank you to former warden David McKune, who granted Elvera Voth permission to start the East Hill Singers and the other arts programming that grew as an outcome of the choir. And deepest gratitude to the faculty in the University of Kansas Music Education and Music Therapy Department, especially my graduate advisor, Dr. James Daugherty, who bolstered my academic skills, challenged my thinking, and guided me into my academic career.

University of Iowa. Multiple people, departments, and groups from the University of Iowa have supported my line of research and this book. Thank you to the Obermann Center for Advanced Studies for awarding me an Obermann Fellowship during my career development leave that included engaging weekly academic conversations as well as space and resources to develop my research. Thank you to Dean Linda Maxson and the Maxson funds; the College Music Society Robby D. Gunstream Education in Music Award; Gene and Priscilla Zimmerman's support of community-engaged research; International Programs' support of my international research travel; the Hazel Prehm Research Assistantships; the College of Education Faculty Research Grant that enabled me to attend the Women's Orchestra Concert inside the Hiland Mountain Correctional Center, Eagle River, Alaska; and the College of Liberal Arts and Sciences Developmental Studies Hybridoma Bank Faculty Scholar award. Thank you to all my departmental executive officers in music (Kristin Thelander, Mark Weiger, David Gier, and Tammie Walker) and the teaching and learning department (Gary Sasso, Peter Hlebowitsh, David Bills, John Hosp, and Lia Plakans) and the remarkable staff in these departments. Thank you to all the administrators and staff in the dean's offices in the College of Education and the College of Liberal Arts and Sciences. Thank you to Adrien Wing and the University of Iowa Center for Human Rights, particularly Dr. Reuben Jonathan Miller's One Community, One Book activities, and Dr. Miller's presentation on his book *Halfway Home: Race, Punishment, and the Afterlife of Mass Incarceration*. Thank you to Jo Butterfield and everyone at the Council for International Visitors to Iowa Cities for your collaboration with the Oakdale Choir. Thank you, Rachel Williams, for your mentorship and scholarly influence. Thank you to the Inside Out Reentry Community for your collaborative work. Thank you to the incredible librarians at the University of Iowa, a partial list of whom includes Janalyn Moss, Paul Soderdahl (and your remarkable musical contributions), Mark Anderson, Willow Fuchs, Katie Buehner, Amy McBeth, Brett Cloyd, Amy Koopmann, and Dan Gall. Thank you to Ryne Carlson for your excellent editorial and indexing work. Thank you to music therapist Kyle Wilhelm who allowed me to accompany him in his work at Oakdale Prison. Thank you to the various students who have provided research assistance, including Willord Simmons, Nathanial Chesher,

Tamara Thies, Joyce Cortesio, Olivia Freesmeier, Calli Hustrulid, Carmen Piedad, Rishi Wagle, and Kristin Conrad. And the numerous students and colleagues who have provided musical leadership with the Oakdale Choir and songwriting workshop including Olivia Freesmeier, Shelly Zeiser, Sean Newman, Chad Clark, Austin Seybert, Rose Schmidt, Annie Savage, James Sherry, Ben Ross, Cinnamon Kleeman, Abby Haywood, Nathaniel De Avila, Lydia Keithley, Karletta White, Haviland Gilbert, Liz Bonnett, Paul Duffy, Joseph Norman, Lori Palamara, Joe Kim, Samuel Raiche, Jonathan Wilson, Alexander Toth, Calli Hustrulid, Giovanna Davila, Simone Frierson, Alisa Kandel, Holly Patch, Jason Palamara, Lori Palamara, Harold Searcy, J. Knight, Kevin B.F. Burt, Murilo Rezende, Matthew Hayes, Connor LaPage, Jane Zhi, Vivien Shotwell, Nancy Menning, Maxine Nash, Suzanne Wedeking, Laura Anderson, Marcy Brant, Kathleen Crose, Megan Felt, Scott Morris, Chris Vinsonhaler, Lauren Katalinich, Tanner Minot, Carolyn Warner, Benjamin Schauer, Isabella DeSoriano, Dana Velthoff, Mitchell Yoon, Lauren Carini, Maryanne Kirsch, Khalda Mohieldin, Duane Warfield, Samuel Cacciatore, Devan Tracey, Macy Schmidt, Tina Freeman, and Chinelo Onuigbo. Thank you to my music education colleagues Jeremy Manternach, Adam Harry, Don Coffman, and Erin Wehr and School of Music and College of Education colleagues, including Courtney Jones, who brought students from his trumpet studio into the Oakdale Prison to perform a composition by University of Iowa alum James Naigus (thank you James!). Thank you to everyone with the University of Iowa Liberal Arts Beyond Bars (UI LABB)—Kathrina Litchfield, Heather Erwin, all the faculty and students who participated, and former University of Iowa president Bruce Harreld. Thanks to so many, many other students who have participated in the Oakdale Choir, graduate seminars on community music, peacebuilding classes, and songwriting workshops, and attended concerts. A special gratitude to Rebecca Swanson for your collaboration on research and musical instruction at Oakdale.

Oakdale Community Choir and the Iowa Department of Corrections. The gratitude story for Oakdale Prison, officially the Iowa Medical and Classification Center, begins with Paula and Lowell Brandt. When I first came to the University of Iowa in the fall of 2007, Paula was my colleague in the College of Education. She ran the Curriculum Library, a remarkable resource for our teacher candidates. Her husband, Lowell, was the Warden at Oakdale Prison. Paula and Lowell sang together, and she encouraged Lowell to meet with me about the idea of starting a choir in the prison. Thanks to his gracious yes, we made plans for an introductory meeting with men in the prison. On December 3, 2008, Lowell died unexpectedly of a heart attack at the age of 58. He was beloved by so many of the men in Oakdale, and by a large community of people who cared for him. His successor, Warden Dan Craig, agreed to continue plans for the February 2009 start of the Oakdale Choir. In addition to Wardens Craig and Brandt, Director of Corrections Jerry Bartruff, Director of the Office of Restorative Justice and Victims Services Mary Roche, and many staff and correctional officers, including Kirsten O'Hare, David Southard, and Adam Drury-Aldrich, worked to accommodate the Oakdale Choir and create additional educational programming, including a Writers' Workshop, Songwriting Workshop, Yoga Class, Job Club, Parenting Class, among others. When Warden Jim McKinney began in October of 2015, the programming expanded, including his collaboration with then-University of Iowa President Bruce Harreld, to initiate UI LABB as mentioned above. Deepest gratitude to Jim McKinney, whose vision of mutual respect, meaningful programming, and tireless collaborative efforts allowed many of the experiences we describe in our book to come to fruition. I have tremendous appreciation for every incarcerated singer and songwriter who stepped into Oakdale Choir rehearsals, stuck with it (even some who mentioned they feared me!), and gave their absolute best—over 175 of you. And tremendous gratitude to each outside singer (over 140 of you), each guest who came into the prison for concerts or other choir events, each student who participated in my Peacebuilding, Singing, and Writing in a Prison Choir class, and Johnathan Kana who collaborated on a writing project as well as graciously donated his lyrics to "Life Within These Walls" and travelled from Texas to attend a concert in the Oakdale Prison—his first visit inside a prison since his release from prison. Thank you to writing and speaking collaborators including Kenneth Bailey, Perry Miller, Arnold Grice, and Richard Winemiller. Gratitude to all the songwriters who gave us permission to use your lyrics in this book. Gratitude to our Oakdale Choir accompanists Linda Stewart Kroon, Joyce Gromko, Colin Kraemer, Allison Schmidt, and Paul Soderdahl. Gratitude to Peter Nothnagle and his excellent audio recording work. Thank you to Tyler Brinegar and your team, who made the Iowa PBS Greetings from Iowa short film about the Oakdale Choir. Thank you to Daniel Kolen and your work on your film *The Inside Singers*. Knowing you would be in rehearsal on any day during the 2015 season improved our focus and rehearsal quality!

Musical influences. The number of musical influences in my life that have impacted this book is tremendous. A short list of the many remarkable people whose work enhances my creative scholarship in this field must include: Melanie DeMore, Maggie Wheeler, Arnae Batson, Barbara McAfee, Debbie Nargi-Brown, Soweto Gospel Choir, Sara Thomsen, Nicholas Payton (especially his "Freedom is No Fear" video with the Music for Abolition series), Terry Lynne Carrington, Vijay Gupta, Yo-Yo Ma, Nimo Patel, Mairi Campbell, Heather Houston, Kim Noller, Dave Camlin, Kristopher Lindquist, Arnold Grice, Ysaye Barnwell, Melissa Ngan, Harold McKinney, the artists on the Die Jim Crow record label, all the musicians in the Oakdale Prison, Eddie Robertson, and my husband, Matt.

Music-making in US prisons colleagues. Again, the number of colleagues who have studied and/or facilitated music-making in US prisons is large and my gratitude runs deep for your inspiring efforts. A partial list includes, with apologies to those I've unintentionally omitted:

Elvera Voth, Catherine Roma, Bea Hasselmann, Meade Palidofsky, Amanda Weber, Jody Kerchner, André de Quadros, Kathryn Hoffer, Kinh Vü, Elliot Cole, Nathan Schram, Eric Shieh, Wayne Kramer, Bill Cleveland, August Tarrier, Fury Young, visual artist and collaborator Jess Perlitz, Kirk Carson, Stephanie Henry, Catherine Wilson, Edward Messerschmidt, Charles Musgrave, Jamey Aebersold, Henry Robinett, Jack Bowers, Wayne Kramer, Jeremy Osborne, Travis Marcum, Megan Holkup, Rebecca Kenaga, Kate Munger, Paula Van Houton, Joe Fierro, Buzzy Martin, Ben Harbert, Sue Coffee, Alex Moroz, Judy Dworin, Laurie Etter, Charlotte White, Laurie Jennings Oudin, Leslie Neal, Judy Bowers, Chaplain Susan Bishop, Jeananne Nichols, Brian Sullivan, Katie Seybert, Maud Hickey, Jason Thompson, Jashen Edwards, Chris Bulgren, Mark Rabideau, Kristina Boerger, Marilyn Knight, Frank Abramson, Eric McIntyre, Heather Herschberger, Jon Cameron, Peggy Forstad, Stephanie Henry, Marles Preheim, Lyle Stutzman, Claire Schwadron, Claudia Frost, Jamie Hillman, Emily Howe, Trey Pratt, Erinn Epp, Randall Speer, Bridget Coughlan Hermer, Bethany Uhler, David Brown, Diana Vuolo, Claire Bryant, Kym Scott, David Osterlund, David McCormick, Mark Gronseth, Mark Edwards, Anne Hamilton, Chaplain Randall Runions, Paul Gambill, David McCormick, Russ Hagen, and with all the artists with Rehabilitation through the Arts, Carnegie Hall Musical Connections, DeCoda Music, HeartBeat Opera (Ethan Heard and Daniel Schlosberg) and all the artists involved in their production of Fidelio, Musicambia, the Creative Arts Program at The Fortune Society, Music on the Inside, other related organizations, and to all my colleagues outside of the US.

Professional influences. Thank you, Lee Willingham, for planning and hosting the 2017 International Community Music Conference at Wilfrid Laurier University (WLU) in Waterloo, Ontario, Canada where the remarkable Senior Editor of WLU Press, Siobhan McMenemy, attended my keynote and afterward contacted me expressing curiosity about a book related to music-making in prisons. Siobhan, thank you for your patience, clear communication, and excellent collaborative nature in the development of this book. Thank you to Murray Tong, Lindsey Hunnewell, Clare Hitchens, all the employees of WLU Press, copy editor Matthew Kudelka, and cover and book designer John van der Woude. Thank you to Jason Chengrian for sharing your painting for the cover art. Thank you to Sabrina Cofer and Bill Mickey with the Authority File Podcast. Thank you to critical and rigorous journalists, including Steve McQueen, Shane Bauer, and Ted Conover. Thank you to all the researchers who have critically examined prisons and abolitionist thinking. The list is too long to include everyone. Some of our influences include Daniel Sered and her work with Common Justice, Carlos Christian, Mariame Kaba, Angela Y. Davis, Ruth Wilson Gilmore, Bettina Love, Maya Schenwar, Victoria Law, Shaka Senghor, Bryan Stevenson, Emily Galvin-Almanza, Elizabeth Hinton, Erica Meiners, Michelle Alexander, Christine Montross, John Pfaff, Derecka Purnell, William Rideau, Fergus McNeill, Shadd Maruna, Hal Pepinsky, Rebecca Ginsburg, Baz Dreisinger, and the thinkers and speakers with the University of Santa Cruz Visualizing Abolition series. Again, the arts-based researchers and groups investigating and practicing in prisons are too long to include everyone. Some of our influences include the organizations Justice Arts Coalition, Arts in Corrections Conferences organized by the William James Association and California Lawyers for the Arts, and individuals Laurie Brooks, Alma Robinson, Larry Brewster, Wendy Jason, Nicole Fleetwood, Ashley Lucas, Curt Tofteland, Mandy Gardner, Grady Hillman, Gregory Sale, Mary Richmiller, Jean Trounstine, and Scott Jackson. Community musicians and educators whose work has influenced us include Gloria Ladson-Billings, Alicia de Banffy-Hall, Kay Pranis, Jennifer Ball, Tahnahga, Kevin Shorner-Johnson, Matthew Thibeault, Olivier Urbain, Natalie Betts, Jennie Henley, Sara Lee, Catherine Birch, Phil Mullen, Lee Higgins, Julie Tiernan, John Speyer, Pete Mosier, Brydie-Leigh Bartleet, Don Coffman, Laya Silber, Andrea Sangiorgio, Alexis Kallio, Graça Mota, Ailbhe Kenny, Inês Lamela,

David Lindsay, Áine Mangaoang, Lukas Pairon, and all the participants of the Social Impact of Making Music research seminar and conferences, the late Bo Lozoff and Buzz Alexander, as well as all of my colleagues with the Community Music Activity Commission of the International Society for Music Education.

We are deeply grateful for everyone who continues to examine critically and explore innovatively how music-making can be a means of building communities of caring. May we each know that within our own hearts we have the seeds to create care for ourselves, our communities, and our planet. Ubuntu. Mitakuye Oyasin. Remember: Be Love.

NOTES

INTRODUCTION

1   This case regarded the legality of the Wisconsin prison authorities removing Juan G. Morales's sister-in-law from his approved correspondence list. This removal was because the social worker intercepted a letter Morales wrote to his sister-in-law, resulting in prison authorities learning that he fathered a child. They assumed that upon his release from prison, while married to his wife, he would continue a relationship with his sister-in-law.

2   Knopp's handbook and the Canadian Quakers' responses sparked the beginning of the International Circle of Penal Abolitionists, which has been meeting biannually since 1983. It is now called the International Conference of Penal Abolitionists. See https://www.justiceaction.org .au/prisons/prison-issues/76-icopa.

3   Bipartisan policies contributed to the mass commutation of the sentences of 500 men and women serving time for low-level drug and theft cases. See Aspinwall 2019.

4   For example, Nancy A. Heitzig argues that police presence in schools criminalizes Blackness while assigning medical labels to white deviance. See Heitzig 2016.

5   The current foster system causes trauma for youth and families. Over 70 percent of siblings are separated, and 36 percent of youth who have aged out of that system experience homelessness. "Think of Us," founded

by former foster youth in 2017, is a research and development lab for child welfare that works to centre people with lived experience in the foster system so as to transform it and provide basic needs for youth and families. See https://www.thinkof-us.org.

6 Corrections Corporation of America, now called CoreCivic, was founded in 1983. It is one of the two largest owners and operators of private detention and correctional facilities in the US. It manages and operates 113 facilities in twenty-two states, including state and federal prisons, immigration detention centres, and jails, and generated US$1.981 billion in revenue in 2021. See https://www.corecivic.com/facilities. Eight percent of prisons in the US are private. GEO Group is the larger of the two private prison companies. These are the only two public real estate investment trusts in the sector. In 2021, both companies suffered a drop in stock prices as a result of pressure from Families Belong Together coalition that included several groups such as MomsRising, Presente.org, Make the Road New York, Little Sis, Real Money Moves, and Interfaith Center on Corporate Responsibility who organized over 600,000 petitions and 500 in-person actions demanding an end to private prison financing. Following these activist efforts, eight major banks, which represented 87.4 percent of private prison financing, stopped financing the industry (Clarke 2021).

7 According to the CoreCivic website, the rebranding included three different business offerings: private prisons (CoreCivic Safety), "government real estate solutions" (CoreCivic Properties), and private re-entry centres (CoreCivic Community). According to the Center for Media and Democracy, in 2013 the Corrections Corporation of America (CCA) employed 15,400 people and made a profit of $300 million based on $1.7 billion in revenue. All of that money came from taxpayers through government contracts. In 2015, CCA contracted out private prisons in eighteen states: Arizona, California, Colorado, Florida, Georgia, Idaho, Indiana, Kentucky, Louisiana, Minnesota, Mississippi, Nevada, New Jersey, New Mexico, Ohio, Oklahoma, Tennessee, and Texas, plus the District of Columbia. As publicly traded companies, CCA and businesses in the same sector such as the GEO Group (which also contracts out with Australia and South Africa, formerly to the United Kingdom), Emerald Correctional Management, and LCS Corrections Services are indebted to their stakeholders and boards of directors,

perhaps more so than they are to the general public and the people who are incarcerated in their facilities. This leads to conflicts of interest with respect to the goals of these companies and the role of justice within the prison system. Many organizations and individuals in the US are now demanding that the ethical issues inherent in the private prison system be addressed. Both companies include "Human Rights Policy" statements on their websites. The CoreCivic statement emphasizes their efforts to prioritize human dignity in their training and daily work (https://www.corecivic.com/hubfs/_files/CoreCivic%20Human%20 Rights%20policy%20statement.pdf). The GEO statement emphasizes respect—first and foremost respect for "the Rule of Law" (https://www .geogroup.com/Portals/0/SR/Human%20Rights/GEO%20Human%20 Rights%20Policy.pdf).

8   These 130 federal facilities include 74 federal correctional medium- and low-security institutions, 23 high-security penitentiaries, 19 administrative facilities in all security categories, 6 federal prison camps, and 8 privately run federal prisons in Texas, Georgia, Oklahoma, and Michigan.

9   Hinton does not examine the Violent Crime Control and Law Enforcement Act, HR 3355, which President Bill Clinton signed into law in 1994. That act provided funding for 100,000 new police officers in addition to $9.7 billion for prisons and $6.1 billion for prevention programs. That act ended access to Pell grants for inmates, which decimated higher education in prisons.

10   It is unlikely that all correctional officers demonstrate the behaviours described by Santos and Rideau, especially given that the US Bureau of Labor Statistics (2020) estimated that 405,870 people work in prisons or jails and that different security protocols exist depending on the security level of the institution. However, institutional rules and protocols continue to hurt people who reside and work behind bars.

11   Efforts toward change are under way. On December 10, 2020, the National Association of Criminal Defense Lawyers released a report, "Second Look = Second Chance," that provided a way for legislatures to safely reduce the number of people serving excessive sentences (Murray et al. 2021).

12   The following countries have recently abolished the death penalty for all crimes: Chad (2020), Burkina Faso (2018), Guinea (2017), Congo, Fiji,

Madagascar, and Suriname (2015), Bolivia (2013), Latvia (2012), Burundi and Togo (2009), Uzbekistan, Chile, and Argentina (2008), Albania and Rwanda (2007), the Philippines (2006), and Liberia and Mexico (2005).

13 Ten people in federal custody, ages 38 to 68, were killed by lethal injection between July and December; another 6 in state custody died by lethal injection; and 1 person (in Tennessee) died by electrocution. See https://deathpenaltyinfo.org/executions/executions-overview/number-of-executions-by-state-and-region-since-1976.

14 The seven founders of the National Deviancy Conference were Kit Carson, Stan Cohen, David Downes, Mary Susan McIntosh, Paul Rock, Ian Taylor, and Jock Young. Its early publications included the edited books *Images of Deviance* (Cohen 1971), *Politics and Deviance: Papers from the National Deviancy Conference* (Taylor and Taylor 1972), and *Contemporary Social Problems in Britain* (Bailey and Young 1973).

15 The many Black peacemakers in the US have included Mary Church Terrell (1863–1954), Addie Waites Hunton (1866–1943), W.E.B. Du Bois (1868–1963), Thurgood Marshall (1908–1993), Shirley Chisholm (1924–2005), and Muhammad Ali (1942–2016). One of many Black musical peacemaking projects related to this book is "Music for Abolition," directed and curated by Terri Lyne Carrington, a collection of sixteen original song compositions with video as part of the University of California, Santa Cruz, Visualizing Abolition webinar series. See https://barringfreedom.org/exhibitions/music-for-abolition.html.

16 Although many of these parents behind bars are mothers, there is a collective shortage of existing scholarship on women's prisons.

17 The Justice Arts Coalition is a US network with resources, programs, events, and a directory of independent arts-based programs in US prisons. See https://thejusticeartscoalition.org.

18 Mary Cohen: I was introduced to music-making in prisons through connections in a Kansas City community choir. Friends in this choir were involved in a not-for-profit organization called Arts in Prison, Inc. (AiP). One Sunday I attended a concert of the East Hill Singers Prison Chorus, supported by AiP. That concert blew my socks off. Men incarcerated at the minimum-security unit of Lansing (Kansas) Correctional Facility travelled to a local church to perform with a chorus of men from the Kansas City area. To see them singing together in unison and harmony, to hear the incarcerated men share narrations

before selections, to see a room full of art created by incarcerated men, and to greet the men after the concert, seeded my curiosity to investigate music education in prisons. Stuart Paul Duncan: I was completing my Doctor of Musical Arts at Cornell University. Doctoral candidates were offered the opportunity to apply to teach a course of their own design at Auburn Correctional Facility, a maximum-security prison, as part of a series of courses that would support incarcerated students in gaining an associate's degree through Cayuga Community College. I had already had the opportunity to work with students who had gone through the traditional route of primary, secondary, then tertiary education; however, the opportunity to experience working with a population who may have not had the same level of access to such an education, or who were returning to an education later in life, was compelling to me. Entering this new educational environment was a daunting and compelling experience for me; it was also profoundly transformative as I came face-to-face with both my own educational privilege and the privilege of being a white male.

19 Throughout this book we use first names when referring to people in custody. Our intention is to contrast this with prisons, which use last names.

20 A few authors have examined the teaching of arts behind bars and have provided introductory material and research related to facilitating musical learning in prisons: Alexander 2010; Anderson 2009; Cheliotis 2012; Cleveland 1992; Martin 2007; Williams 2003.

21 "Healing Justice" is the name of a national not-for-profit organization supporting people who have experienced inequity and trauma in the US. See https://healingjusticeproject.org. It is also the title of a book by Loretta Pyles.

CHAPTER 1

1 Many researchers have tested this theory. For example, see Messerschmidt 2017; Thompson 2016; Wilson 2013; and Doxat-Pratt (2018).

2 The Liz Lerman Critical Response Process is a four-step strength-based process that starts with positive feedback and then allows the artist to ask the responders questions about their work. Step three involves neutral

questions from the responders, and the final step includes opportunities for responders to share their opinions with the artist.

3   The audio recordings from concerts were originally in the form of compact discs. Many recordings are also available digitally on the Oakdale Choir website. See http://oakdalechoir.lib.uiowa.edu.

4   The facility's warden decides on the level of engagement between guests and choir members. For example, when the Oakdale Choir began, we scheduled concerts for outside guests on Wednesdays so that family members could spend the night in the area and have a visit on Thursday. Visiting days at this prison were Thursday through Sunday. Inside singer Arnold Grice requested approval to have a visit before a concert. After this concert, where chairs were set up around the edges of the gym, the prison administrators decided it would be easier to move the concerts to Thursdays so that the visits occurred on an actual visiting day. When Jim McKinney worked as warden from 2015 to 2020, he allowed larger audiences, up to 300 people, and we moved concerts to Saturdays so that more family members could travel to the prison for the events.

5   Electronic communication in prisons is different than email outside of prisons. There are limits on characters, security staff members review the messages, and data retention policies are different than traditional email systems.

CHAPTER 2

1   This quote by van de Wall resonates closely with the South African concept, *Ubuntu*, which is a core component of the Oakdale Prison Community Choir in Iowa.

2   In his ninety-page report, he noted several key problems: first, lack of training for staff and administrators; second, state governors who appoint unqualified wardens; third, labour issues in prisons; fourth, thirty- to forty-year sentences, compared to one- to five-year sentences in England or Germany. When responding to the question of whether there were facts that would indicate a "soft-hearted" and "coddling" treatment of people in prison, he wrote: "*to the mind of the European, an often shocking brutality is characteristic of American criminal procedures and of American prisons*" (p. 16), including the execution of a young man at nineteen years

old and a sixteen-year-old boy in Sing Sing Prison (New York). According to the Equal Justice Initiative, racial terror lynchings included 4,084 African American men, women, and children between 1877 and 1950 in twelve southern states, and 300 racial terror lynchings in other states. Youth executions, as horrific as they are, similar to these lynchings, were part of white domination. See https://lynchinginamerica.eji.org/report/.

3 Although it is beyond the scope of this project to examine all music programs in US prisons in the twentieth century, the programs selected provide a broad array for review.

4 According to Sporny (1941), in 1940–41, Boston University began offering a course to prepare people to facilitate music informally for social purposes. Sporny quoted from the Boston University catalogue: "Fundamental value of music in social and personal adjustment. Methods and technique for the use of music in informal groups. Correlation of music with other phases of recreational programs, with drama and dance" (8–9). With respect to Sporny's findings regarding the institutional instructors' musical training, some teachers have earned an AB or BS degree and two of them a master's degree. The rest are graduates from Sacred Heart Mission, the US School of Music in Chicago, the Leipzig Conservatory in Germany, and Fontainbleau Conservatory in France. Those with no musical degrees have a wide range of backgrounds including private instruction on their instrument, a few years playing experience, and retired Marine and Army musicians (7). Sporny specifically noted: "We find music teachers not very well qualified or prepared" (7).

5 Forty-five of the sixty-nine institutions that responded to his survey (encompassing twenty-four states as well as Washington, DC) indicated they had bands ranging in size from 9 to 100 people; 40 had orchestras ranging from 9 to 25 men (21), and around 30 offered music appreciation classes.

6 These states were Alabama, Colorado, Connecticut, Delaware, Florida, Idaho, and Michigan (Hodson 1951, 40–81).

7 A summary of Apicella's findings: 10 percent of the institutions that returned the survey reported no music activities; 30 percent offered only a few music activities; and 87.9 percent of the penal institutions that returned the questionnaire provided music activities where the incarcerated individuals performed or listened. All institutions for individuals experiencing mental illness provided recorded music over a public address system, and some administrators stated that "music is

effective in soothing and relaxing the emotionally disturbed individuals" (82).

8   Landreville (1956) sent questionnaires inquiring about music activities, equipment, personnel, finances, and general information. He focused on the following states in the US Northwest—Washington, Oregon, Idaho, Wyoming, and Montana—and on federal prisons in California, Kansas, Indiana, Pennsylvania, and Georgia.

9   Note the referencing of Willem van de Wall.

10   Littell was a graduate student at the University of Kansas who studied with E. Thayer Gaston, a psychologist who contributed to music therapy research. Our research in this book does not include a thorough examination of music therapy in prisons. More study in this area is warranted.

11   Littell's response rate was 60 percent. Of the 197 completed surveys, 94.4 percent reported using music in their facilities. Funding for 69.5 percent of these programs was through budgeted appropriations; 71.1 percent of the facilities stated that their music programs were inadequate because of the lack of finances and properly trained personnel. The top seven musical activities in these prisons were choir, talent shows, band, instrumental instruction, music appreciation, vocal instruction, and dance band.

12   Categories for "other" included religious services only, rodeo, outlet for musicians, public relations, academic training, music appreciation, and religious training.

13   Littell's data collection focused on the following four points: the use and purpose of music in correctional institutions, the characteristics of personnel in the music program, the nature of musical activities, and additional remarks. His goal was to ascertain whether correctional institutions were suitable venues for music therapists and whether they would need modifications of or additional courses in their academic training.

14   Also in 1954, the organization changed its name from the American Prison Association to the American Correctional Association.

15   The fifth point in the 1954 ACA Declaration of Principles states: "The prisoner's destiny should be placed in his own hands; he must be put into circumstances where he will be able, through his own exertions, to continually better his own condition. A regulated self-interest must be brought into play, and made constantly operative." ACA 1954, 409.

16 The Wisconsin Department of Corrections states 1908 as the year the prison band began. See https://doc.wi.gov/Pages/AboutDOC/DepartmentHistory.aspx.

17 Among other reforms, the dungeons were closed and corporal punishment was ended. Warden Duffy abandoned gun towers, desegregated the dining hall, and improved the prison food. He also started a new weekly hobby program that enabled incarcerated men to earn money, opened a canteen to reduce gambling and contraband trade, opened an Alcoholics Anonymous chapter, and started a prison newspaper.

18 This approach to training horses is now widely regarded as cruel. Given the well-established link between cruelty to animals and crimes against other people, this type of "rehabilitation" program is no longer something to celebrate.

19 Chaplain Grandstaff, the director of The Prodigals in the Missouri Training Center for Men in the 1960s, recalled: "In some of those small towns, where they hadn't even seen many Blacks, it was a little scary, and they were somewhat anxious. But before the night was over, you didn't know who was who. At first, we put whites with whites, and blacks with blacks. But we eventually altered that too. And we'd put a black inmate with a white family, and so forth. But usually before the night was over, everyone was laughing and having a wonderful time. And that was another milestone and we'd broken ground in a new place. I'd run over to the piano after they'd eaten and strike a chord or two on the piano, and the guys all knew it. So they'd start singing the opening number from where they were sitting. It just chokes you up to remember it. There were guys from all over the dining room coming up to sing. It was just great. People loved it. The guys were dressed in white shirts and ties. So they weren't sitting there in stripes, but that was the conventional view of the inmate … I had to work with each inmate when he came into the choir. He had to have the confidence in himself before he was ready to go out." Qtd in Richmiller 1992, 101.

CHAPTER 3

1 In his first year, Jack Bowers was a contract teacher for the William James Association. The second year he was a California Arts Council Artist in Residence. The third year he was the Education Department Music

Teacher, and the remainder of the time (through 2007) he was the Institution Artist Facilitator with the Arts in Corrections Program. Email correspondence with Mary Cohen, December 3, 2021.

2   Another longstanding instrumental music educator in prisons was Mark Edwards, who facilitated instrumental and vocal music learning for men in the State Correctional Institution – Graterford in Pennsylvania from 1983 to 2005. Edwards was employed full-time by the Pennsylvania Department of Corrections, and he indicated there were eight or nine full-time music teachers in Pennsylvania while he was teaching.

3   Jamey Aebersold gave instruments, instrument guides, books, and records to people in many prisons, including in Alabama, Arizona, California, Illinois, Indiana, Kentucky, Massachusetts, New Mexico, New York, Oklahoma, Ohio, and Tennessee, and he remains in touch with currently and formerly incarcerated musicians (Shouse 2021; personal correspondence, January 1, 2022).

4   McCarty and Brayboy (2021), among others, describe extensions of culturally relevant pedagogy, including culturally based education, culturally responsive schooling, and culturally sustaining and revitalizing pedagogies (CSRP). CSRP, they note, focuses on perspectives, experiences, and contributions created in Native American/Indigenous education contexts.

5   More than 30 percent of the world's incarcerated women are in the US, although only 4 percent of the world's women live there (Dallaire and Poehlmann-Tynan 2021, 3). Yet there has been very little research on music-making in US women's prisons.

6   See https://artsontheedge.weebly.com; and McCoy 2012.

7   Each December the women at Hiland adopt a family and purchase gifts for them using proceeds from the sales of their crafts such as bags, backpacks, hats, scarves, and quilts. People who come into the prison for the orchestra concert purchase these items.

8   Compare this to Norway, where the music provisions in forty-two different prisons in 2019 were funded by the government.

9   The November 30, 2018, earthquake near Anchorage required the staff to cancel the concert of December 1, 2018. The damage to the facility could not be ascertained until the snow melted and a thorough inspection was possible. There was less damage than expected. The Hiland Orchestra's performance of Nancy Strelau's "The Journey" was the highlight of the

December 2019 concert. The women wrote about their own journeys and read portions of their thank you notes to Strelau at the concert. Strelau was the orchestra director of the New York All State Orchestra in 2019 and was unable to travel to Anchorage for the premiere of her piece. She plans to have it published with all income from its sales donated to Hiland. Strelau first learned about Hiland when she met Hoffer through a mutual friend at the American String Teachers Association annual conference.

10 Their first five pieces were "Serenata," *New World Symphony*, "Eagles on Air," "Twinkle Little Star," and "Are You Sleeping?"

CHAPTER 4

1   These are select themes from Oakdale Choir concerts. See http://oakdalechoir.lib.uiowa.edu/category/performance.

2   For more findings about on masculinity in prisons, see Sabo, Kuper, and London 2001; and Maycock and Hunt 2019.

3   When Mary Cohen checked in with Tom twelve years later, he noted that what he wrote about his separation from his wife back in 2009 "goes double for now." He explained that it does not matter how long someone is in prison, a part of them yearns for the family and friends that have been lost.

4   For example, in 2012 Roma co-founded the World House Choir with Reverend Derrick Weston, Director of the Coretta Scott King Center at Antioch College. The name "World House Choir" comes from a reflection by Martin Luther King, Jr., who said we have all inherited our modern world, and it is a house in which we must live together: "We have inherited a large house, a great 'world house' in which we have to live together—black and white, Easterner and Westerner, Gentile and Jew, Catholic and Protestant, Moslem and Hindu—a family unduly separated in ideas, culture, and interest, who, because we can never again live apart, must learn somehow to live with each other in peace" (King 1967, 167). See https://worldhousechoir.org.

5   Charities that have received financial support from Roma's incarcerated singers include Word Play, Cincinnati (https://www.wordplaycincy .org); Artemis Center: Dayton's Domestic Violence Resource Agency

(https://artemiscenter.org); CAIN: Churches Active in Northside (http://www.cainministry.org); and Local Matters (https://www .local-matters.org).

6　　There were 7,530 minutes of choral performance in these games. Medals awarded included 106 gold, 139 silver, and 19 bronze. See https://www .interkultur.com/events/world-choir-games/cincinnati-2012.

7　　See https://www.interkultur.com/events/world-choir-games/ cincinnati-2012. The book is titled *Share Song. Create Magic. Capturing the Memories of the 2012 World Choir Games, World Choir Games 2012 Cincinnati, USA*. See Interkultur video: https://www.youtube.com/ watch?v=FptOztQbK-o. An important consideration here is that survivors of crime may feel traumatized by the incarcerated singers' success. The National Center for Victims of Crime and various other state and local programs provide resources for crime victims.

8　　Ear Hustle is a podcast out of San Quentin State Prison in California that comments on the daily realities of prison life for people incarcerated there as well as stories of post-incarceration life. See https://www .earhustlesq.com.

　　　Three additional podcasts from people inside US prisons are prisonradio.org, weareuncuffed.org, and Prison Prophets (https:// www.songsinthekeyoffree.com/prison-prophets-podcast). Prison Radio broadcasts examine issues that create crime and disenfranchise communities and their educational materials intend to generate public activism and build movements for social change. Uncuffed is based out of California prisons, and Prison Prophets is from a maximum security prison in Montgomery County, Pennsylvania. Additionally, Inside Wire is a 24 hour Colorado Prison Radio Program that began in 2022. See http://www.coloradoprisonradio.com/. For a critical and historical discussion of a weekly radio program that started in 1938 and ran over five years, planned by Texas State Prison authorities and aimed to positively influence the public, see Ethan Blue (2012) "Thirty Minutes behind the Walls" in *Doing Time in the Depression: Everyday Life in Texas and California Prisons*.

9　　Catherine Roma has created "choral communities of healing, hope, and love" in a hostile environment: see Roma 2018, 28. Having had a strong Quaker education, she has infused Quaker tenets such as engaged activism, peacebuilding, equal consideration of all people, and a communal model of decision-making into her musical practices and life. *Ubuntu* is a South African term meaning "we are who we are through our relationship with others."

10　See https://www.wilmington.edu/mata.

11　See https://www.ohioprisonartsconnection.org. Other Ohio prison choir leaders are Dr. Jody Kerchner, founder and leader of the Oberlin College and Grafton Correctional Institution Choir, whose college students participate in prison education projects; and David Brown, founder and leader of the Harmony Project in partnership with Tapestry at the Ohio Reformatory for Women. Brown's program includes an inside/outside choir, and incarcerated choir members sometimes participate in outside performances with a live feed via computer screen. See https://www.harmonyproject.com.

12　See https://www.healingbrokencircles.org.

13　*Ubuntu* is also the name of the choir Roma founded at London Correctional Institution and the grounding framework for the Oakdale Choir in Iowa.

14　In addition to "Let's Go Make History" (https://vimeo.com/239149484), the OJPC anniversary celebration included the KUJI Men's Chorus singing Guy Banks's "Anybody Out There" (https://vimeo.com/239149266) and HOPE Thru Harmony's Women's Chorus singing Carolyn Maillard's "The Women Gather" (https://vimeo.com/240684880). Alphonse Gerhardstein founded the Ohio Justice and Policy Center in 1997; in 2015, he went in front of the Supreme Court to argue for marriage equality and won.

15　The size of the full chorus fluctuated throughout the history of this choir between fifty and eighty men. The Lansing administrators decided whether the person in custody could leave the prison for concerts or not.

16　Arts in Prison, Inc., offers a wide variety of arts programming inside the Lansing Correctional Facility, including writing, theatre, yoga and meditation, public speaking, visual arts, knitting, and crochet. See www.artsinprison.org.

17　Kirk Carson continued to lead the East Hill Singers from 2008 through 2018; he was followed by Dr. Joseph Kern on an interim basis until 2020. Other performing arts programs that have begun at Lansing through Arts in Prison, Inc., are Living Shakespeare, Spoken Word, and Improvisation.

18 All graduate students were required to participate, and other members had the option to participate. For applications of this reflective writing component for other musical ensembles, see Mary L. Cohen 2012c.

19 See the link to past newsletters, with excerpts from the reflective writing exchange, under the link "Press": http://oakdalechoir.lib.uiowa.edu/.

20 Two additional courses were a yoga class and a University of Iowa Faculty Series course with different topics each week. The faculty series was designed to introduce many different faculty members to teaching in a prison and the idea of college to the men in the prison. The yoga class shifted from a credit-bearing course to a weekly guided practice with three different volunteer yoga instructors. These courses stopped when Covid-19 eliminated volunteer programs.

21 Melanie DeMore is a vocal activist based in Oakland, California. She composed "Lead with Love" the day after the 2016 US presidential election. See http://www.melaniedemore.com.

22 The choirs were UBUNTU, KUJI, HOPE thru Harmony, Voices of Hope, the East Hill Singers, and the Oakdale Choir. See https://www.youtube.com/watch?v=J_ipFPVLUS8 for a summary of this project and https://www.youtube.com/watch?v=x5O1fBAnhvo for the premiere performance of "O welche Lust." HeartBeat Opera completed a virtual album called *Breathing Free* in 2020 and toured *Fidelio* with video and audio recordings of these incarcerated singers in spring 2022.

23 Due to Covid-19, the choir season and Peacebuilding Class shifted abruptly. The Oakdale Choir's last rehearsal and class in the prison was March 3, 2020. Then the outside choir rehearsed virtually using Zoom. We recorded our rehearsals and shared the audio files with the technology supervisor at the prison, asking him to share the files with the men at Oakdale. We provided audio practice files for the men to listen to on their own. We concluded the season with a virtual "Listening Exchange" in May, with recordings of the Oakdale Choir from past performances and some original written reflections and visual art from incarcerated students in the Peacebuilding Class.

24 See https://www.facebook.com/TheInsideSingers.

25 MUSE is an acronym for Musical excellence, Unity, Social justice, and Empowerment. In Greek and Roman mythology, the muses were the nine daughters of Zeus and Mnemosyne and presided over the arts and sciences. The term also means a person or personified force who inspires creative artists.

CHAPTER 5

1   In one recent study, respondents who read poetry about currently incarcerated individuals' childhoods held significantly less stigma toward formerly incarcerated people compared to respondents who read about recidivism. See Dum 2021.

2   Perhaps a plan could be developed whereby someone or an organization commissioned musical arrangements or compositions and then paid incarcerated musicians' families for those creations; however, huge complexities exist regarding publishing, administration, and financial details. The organization Jail Guitar Doors began in 2007 in the UK when Billy Bragg received a request from Malcolm Dudley, who had started a guitar class while working as a drug and alcohol counsellor at HMP Guys Marsh in Dorset, England. Bragg established JGD in honour of Joe Strummer, a founding member of The Clash, a British punk rock band. JGD provides instruments and musical instruction to more than twenty prisons in the UK. Wayne and Margaret Saadi Kramer partnered with Bragg to launch Jail Guitar Doors USA in 2009. The Kramers and their team have also built Community Arts Programming and Outreach (CAPO) for youth in Los Angeles County probation camps and released from juvenile halls. They are working with the Los Angeles County Library to release recordings these youths create (personal correspondence, September 24, 2021). See https://www.jailguitardoors .org.uk/ and https://jail-guitar-doors.myshopify.com..

3   For example, we were learning songs such as "Homeward Bound," "Sometimes I Feel Like a Motherless Child," and "Ose Shalom."

4   The first verse and chorus of Kenneth Bailey's "Crossroads" are as follows:

> There are moments in your life
> when you need to make a choice
> as the crossroads are pressing down on you.
>
> Leave the fears you have behind
> as you take a step ahead.
> For no one ever knows
> just how it all will end.

CHORUS
Go, Go! Move onward with your life
sometimes left and sometimes right.
Let the heart that guides your love
guide your days and guide your nights.
Then your crossroads will never be mistakes.

5   In the first season of the choir, we used Stephen King's (2000) memoir
    On Writing, and the writing prompts were based on ideas about the
    similarities and differences between singing and writing. I (Cohen)
    taught a graduate seminar in conjunction with the first season, and all
    graduate students sang in the choir and were required to participate in
    the writing exchange. For the third choir season we used *We're All Doing
    Time* by Bo Lozoff and for the fourth season, *Musicking: The Meanings of
    Performing and Listening* by Christopher Small. Other seasons the writing
    prompts were based on lyrics of the songs we sang, seasonal topics, and
    other choir-related reflections.

6   Mary Trachsel, a University of Iowa professor and charter outside singer
    of the Oakdale Choir, started a weekly Writers' Workshop at Oakdale in
    August 2009. Kenneth Bailey participated in that workshop from its start
    until he was transferred to another facility.

7   See https://www.storycatcherstheatre.org.

8   See https://www.youtube.com/watch?v=NygVs60LaYA&list=PLyS59q
    N9ygL2tvUO4LKM4Wkwb2hwrUgWg.

9   Another musical resource for children whose parents are incarcerated
    is Scaling Walls a Note at a Time (SWAN), which provides free music
    education for these youth. See https://swan4kids.org.

10 Premiered at the December 2011 concert themed "Winds of Change."

11 Recordings of these new spirituals have been captured on CDs. Twenty-
    nine original songs composed by the choir members are on four CDs,
    three of them created with UMOJA ("Feel Like, Going On," "Do It for
    the Children," "Extend a Hand") and one with UBUNTU ("Begin to
    Love"). Upon examination of some of Alan Lomax's field recordings
    from Mississippi State Penitentiary—most often referred to as Parchman
    Farm—in 1947–48, as well as examine the research that Alan and his
    father John had conducted in 1933. The Lomaxes thought they would
    collect the oldest African American songs, but instead, they collected

original repertoire that the men in custody sang while doing heavy labour on chain gangs. The songs "are a vivid reminder of a system of social control and forced labor that has endured in the South for centuries; and I do not believe that the pattern of Southern life can be fundamentally reshaped until what lies behind these roaring, iconic choruses is understood" (*Prison Songs*, 1997; see also *The Southern Journey of Alan Lomax: Words, Photographs, and Music*, 2013).

12 The score is available on the compilation of original musical compositions by Roma's prison choir members, "Songs of Freedom and Resilience." The Ohio Voices for Justice created a recording of "Black Lives Matter." See https://www.youtube.com/watch?v=A2TTVzzyBdM.

13 See https://www.youtube.com/watch?v=A2TTVzzyBdM.

14 See https://www.diejimcrow.com.

15 See https://www.songsinthekeyoffree.com.

16 See https://prisonprophets.captivate.fm.

17 See https://www.songsinthekeyoffree.com/about.

18 See https://www.easternstate.org/explore/artist-installations/jess-perlitz-chorus.

19 See https://barringfreedom.org/exhibitions/music-for-abolition.html.

CHAPTER 6

1 Rebecca Ginsburg is the founder of the Education Justice Project, a comprehensive college-in-prison program based at the University of Illinois Urbana-Champaign. See https://educationjustice.net/about.

2 Susan D. Blum (2020) and thirteen other researchers explore pedagogical and practical aspects of "ungrading."

3 Many support systems for re-entry have been not-for-profit, community-based systems such as Inside Out Reentry. See https://www.insideoutreentry.com.

4 He specifically referenced Emile Durkheim, Arnold van Gennep, Mary Douglas, Kai Erikson, Thomas Scheff, John Braithwaite, and Randall Collins.

5 The 13th Amendment, "Neither slavery nor involuntary servitude, *except as a punishment for crime whereof the party shall have been duly convicted*, shall exist within the United States, or any place subject to

their jurisdiction" (emphasis added), allows for enslaved labour inside US prisons.

6   As performed by Arnold Grice and the Oakdale Choir in Spring 2012. See http://oakdalechoir.lib.uiowa.edu/original-works.

WORKS CITED

ACA (American Correctional Association). 1954. *Manual of Correctional Standards*. 303, 3rd ed.

Alexander, Buzz. 2010. *Is William Martinez Not Our Brother? Twenty Years of the Prison Creative Arts Project*. Ann Arbor: University of Michigan Press.

Alexander, Michelle. 2010. *The New Jim Crow: Mass Incarceration in the Age of Colorblindness*. New York: New Press.

American Journal of Correction. 1956. "Résumé of the 86th Annual Congress of Correction." 8, no. 5 (September–October): 8–14, 20–29.

Anderson, Kirstin. 2009. *Teaching Music in Prisons: Introductory Information and Ideas for Musicians and Teachers Working in Prisons*. Edinburgh: Institute for Music in Human and Social Development at the University of Edinburgh.

Apicella, Anthony. 1952. "A Survey of Music Activities in the Penal Institutions of Northeastern United States." MA thesis, Boston University.

Aspinwall, Cary. 2019. "How More Than 50 Women Walked Out of a Prison in Oklahoma: The State Slashed Sentences for More than 500 People Convicted in Low-Level Drug and Theft Cases," 4 November. The Marshall Project. https://www.themarshallproject.org/2019/11/04/how-more-than-50-women-walked-out-of-a-prison-in-oklahoma.

Bailey, Roy Victor, and Jock Young, eds. 1973. *Contemporary Social Problems in Britain*. Farnborough: Saxon House.

Bauer, Shane. 2018. *American Prison: A Reporter's Undercover Journey into the Business of Punishment*. New York: Penguin Books.

Blue, Ethan. 2012. *Doing Time in the Depression: Everyday Life in Texas and California Prisons*. Oxford University Press.

Blum, Susan. D., ed. 2020. *Ungrading: Why Rating Students Undermines Learning (and What to Do Instead)*. Morgantown: West Virginia University Press.

Boal, Augusto. 1985. *Theatre of the Oppressed*. Translated by Charles A. and Maria-Odilia Leal McBride. New York: Theatre Communications Group.

———. 2006. *The Aesthetics of the Oppressed*. Translated by Adrian Jackson. New York: Routledge.

Bronston, Jennifer, and Marcus Berzofsky. 2017. "Indicators of Mental Health Problems Reported by Prisoners and Jail Inmates, 2011–2012." Washington, DC: US Department of Justice, Bureau of Justice Statistics.

Brubaker, Mike. 2014. "Prisoner #7290 A Lifer in Music." *TempoSenzaTempo*. 8 August. http://temposenzatempo.blogspot.com/2014/08/prisoner-7280-lifer-in-music.html.

Bulgren, Christopher W. 2020. "Jail Guitar Doors: A Case Study of Guitar and Songwriting Instruction in Cook County Jail." *International Journal of Community Music* 13, no. 3: 299–318.

Canadian Yearly Meeting of the Religious Society of Friends. 1981. "Minute on Prison Abolition." Minute 93. https://quakerservice.ca/wp-content/uploads/2011/05/cym-Minute-on-Prison-Abolition.pdf.

Carnes, Aaron. 2017. "Jailhouse Blues: Henry Robinett on Teaching Inmates to Play the Guitar." *The Sun*, October, 6–13.

Carson, E. Ann. 2021. "Prisoners in 2020 – Statistical Tables." Washington, DC: US Department of Justice, NCJ 302776. December. https://bjs.ojp.gov/library/publications/prisoners-2020-statistical-tables.

Cary, C.P. 1910. *14th Biennial Report of the Wisconsin State Prison*, 30 June. Madison.

Casella, Jean, James Ridgeway, and Sarah Shourd. 2016. *Hell Is a Very Small Place: Voices from Solitary Confinement*. New York: New Press.

Casey, Betty Jo, Kim Taylor-Thompson, Estée Rubien-Thomas, Maria Robbins, and Arielle Baskin-Sommers. 2020. "Healthy Development as a Human Right: Insights from Developmental Neuroscience for Youth Justice." *Annual Review of Law and Social Science* 16: 203–22.

Cheliotis, Leonidas K., ed. 2012. *The Arts of Imprisonment: Control, Resistance, and Empowerment*. Burlington: Ashgate.

Chipungu, Sandra Stukes, and Tricia B. Bent-Goodley. 2004. "Meeting the Challenges of Contemporary Foster Care." *The Future of Children* 14, no. 1: 74–93.

CLA (California Lawyers for the Arts). n.d. "Arts in Corrections National Conference." https://www.calawyersforthearts.org/arts-in-corrections .html.

Clarke, Matthew. 2021. "Private Prison Companies Face Stock Crash, Credit Crunch." *Prison Legal News*, 1 February 2021, 40.

Clements-Cortés, Amy. 2015. "Clinical Effects of Choral Singing for Older Adults." *Music and Medicine* 7, no. 4: 7–12.

Cleveland, William. 1992. *Art in Other Places: Artists at Work in America's Community and Social Institutions.* Westport: Praeger.

Cohen, Mary L. 2007a. "Christopher Small's Concept of Musicking: Toward a Theory of Choral Singing Pedagogy in Prison Contexts." PhD diss., University of Kansas.

———. 2007b. "Explorations of Inmate and Volunteer Choral Experiences in a Prison-Based Choir." *Australian Journal of Music Education* 1: 61–72.

———. 2008a (March). "'I Wish I Never Hurt You': Select Texts and Contexts of Prison Choirs." Lecture, Cultural Diversity in Music Education Conference, Seattle.

———. 2008b. "'Mother Theresa, How Can I Help You?' The Story of Elvera Voth, Robert Shaw, and the Bethel College Benefit Sing-Along for Arts in Prison, Inc." *International Journal of Research in Choral Singing* 3, no. 1: 4–22.

———. 2009. "Conductors' Perspectives of Kansas Prison Choirs." *International Journal of Community Music* 1, no. 3 (2009): 319–33.

———. 2012a. "Harmony within the Walls: Perceptions of Worthiness and Competence in a Prison Choir." *International Journal of Music Education* 30, no. 1: 47–57.

———. 2012b. "Safe Havens: The Formation and Practice of Prison Choirs in the US." In *The Arts of Imprisonment: Control, Resistance, and Empowerment*, edited by Leonidas K. Cheliotis, 227–34. Farnham: Ashgate.

———. 2012c. "Writing between Rehearsals: A Tool for Assessment and Building Camaraderie." *Music Educators Journal* 98, no. 3: 43–48. doi:10.1177/0027432111434743.

———. 2019a. "As Far As the Ear Can Hear: Choral Singing in Prisons Grows a Community of Caring." In *As Far As the Eye Can See: The Promises and Perils of Research and Scholarship in the 21st Century*, edited by Stephen J. Pradarelli, 141–48. Iowa City: University of Iowa Press.

———. 2019b. "Choral Singing in Prisons: Evidence Based Practices to Support Returning Citizens." *Prison Journal 99*, no. 4: 106S–117S.

Cohen, Mary L., and Stuart Paul Duncan. 2015. "Restorative and Transformative Justice and Its Relationship to Music Education within and beyond Prison Contexts." In *The Oxford Handbook of Social Justice in Music Education*, edited by Cathy Benedict, Patrick Schmidt, Gary Spruce, and Paul Woodford, 554–66. New York: Oxford University Press.

Cohen, Mary L., and Jennie Henley. 2018. "Music-Making behind Bars: The Many Dimensions of Community Music in Prisons." In *The Oxford Handbook of Community Music*, edited by Brydie-Leigh Bartleet and Lee Higgins, 153–76. Oxford: Oxford University Press.

Cohen, Mary L., Johnathan Kana, and Richard Winemiller. 2021. "Life within These Walls: Community Music-Making as a Bridge of Healing and Transformation in Prison Contexts." In *Community Music at the Boundaries*, edited by Lee Willingham, 383–401. Waterloo: Wilfrid Laurier University Press.

Cohen, Mary L., and Meade Palidofsky. 2013. "Changing Lives: Incarcerated Female Youth Create and Perform with the Storycatchers Theatre and the Chicago Symphony Orchestra." *American Music 31*, no. 3: 163–82.

Cohen, Mary L., and Catherine Wilson. 2017. "Inside the Fences: The Processes and Purposes of Songwriting in an Adult Male Prison." *International Journal of Music Education 35*, no. 4: 543–51.

Cohen, Stanley, ed. 1971. *Images of Deviance*. London: Penguin Books.

Coleman, Wayland "X." 2020. "Remember Me for the Love That I Have in Me." In *My Body Was Left on the Street: Music Education and Displacement*, edited by Kinh T. Vü and André de Quadros, 100–101. Boston: Brill.

Common Justice. n.d. "The Common Justice Model." https://www.commonjustice.org/the_common_justice_model.

"CoreCivic, Inc. Form 10-K for Fiscal Year Ended December 31, 2017." EDGAR. Securities and Exchange Commission, 2018, https://www.sec.gov/Archives/edgar/data/1070985/000156459018002898/cxw-10k_20171231.htm

Cozart, Reed. 1956a. "Citizen Participation in the South." *American Journal of Correction 18*, no. 5 (September–October): 27.

———. 1956b. "Coordinating Treatment in the Total Correctional Process." *American Journal of Correction 18*, no. 5 (September–October): 24.

Cursley, Jo, and Shadd Maruna. 2015. "A Narrative-Based Evaluation of 'Changing Tunes' Music-Based Prisoner Reintegration Interventions:

Full Report." January. Arts Alliance Evidence Library. http://www
.artsevidence.org.uk/evaluations/narrative-based-evaluation-changing
-tunes-music-ba/.

Dallaire, Danielle H., and Julie Poehlmann-Tynan. 2021. "Introduction
to Incarcerated Mothers and their Children: Separation, Loss, and
Reunification." In *Children with Incarcerated Mothers: Separation, Loss,
and Reunification,* edited by Julie Poehlmann-Tynan and Danielle H.
Dallaire, 1–11. New York: Springer.

Datchi, Corinne C., and Julie R. Ancis, eds. 2017. "Gender, Psychology, and
Justice: The Mental Health of Women and Girls in the Legal System." In
Psychology and Crime Series, 2. New York: NYU Press.

de Quadros, André. 2015. "Rescuing Choral Music from the Realm of the
Elite: Models for Twenty-First Century Music Making – Two Case
Illustrations." In *The Oxford Handbook of Social Justice in Music Education,*
edited by Cathy Benedict, Patrick Schmidt, Gary Spruce, and Paul
Woodford, 501–12. Oxford: Oxford University Press.

———. 2016. "Case Study: 'I once was lost but now am found' – Music and
Embodied Arts in Two American Prisons." In *Oxford Textbook of Creative
Arts, Health, and Wellbeing: International Perspectives on Practice, Policy,
and Research,* edited by Stephen Clift and P.M. Camic, 187–91. New York:
Oxford University Press.

———. 2018. "Community Music: Portraits of Struggle, Identity, and
Togetherness." In *The Oxford Handbook of Community Music,* edited
by Brydie-Leigh Bartleet and Lee Higgins, 266–80. New York: Oxford
University Press.

———. 2019. *Choral Music in Global Perspective.* New York: Routledge.

de Quadros, André, and Emilie Amrein. 2023 (forthcoming). *Empowering
Song: Music Education from the Margins.* Routledge.

Death Penalty Information Center. n.d. "Executions Overview." https://
deathpenaltyinfo.org/executions/executions-overview.

Denhof, Michael D., Caterina G. Spinaris, and Gregory R. Morton. 2014.
"Occupational stressors in corrections organizations: Types, effects, and
solutions." http://nicic.gov/library/028299.

Douglas, Andy. 2019. *Redemption Songs: A Year in the Life of a Community
Prison Choir.* San Germán: InnerWorld.

Doxat-Pratt, Sarah. 2018. "Changing the Record: Reassessing Effectiveness and
Value in Prison Music Projects." PhD diss., University of Nottingham.

Doyle, James. 1972. *Morales v. Schmidt* 340 Federal Supplement. W.D. Wis 1972. 544, 548–59.

Duffy, Clinton T., and Dean Jennings. 1968. *The San Quentin Story.* New York: Greenwood Press.

Dum, Christopher P., Kelly M. Socia, Bengt George, and Halle M. Neiderman. 2021. "The Effect of Reading Prisoner Poetry on Stigma and Public Attitudes: Results from a Multigroup Survey Experiment." *The Prison Journal.* https://doi.org/10.1177/00328855211069127.

Duncan, Stuart P. 2013. "Moving beyond Disciplinary Boundaries: Transformative Aspects of Contract Grading and Pedagogy." *Yale Teaching Center* (blog), 17 October. http://yalegtc.blogspot.com/2013/10/moving-beyond-disciplinary-boundaries.html.

Duwe, Grant, and Byron R. Johnson. 2016. "The Effects of Prison Visits from Community Volunteers on Offender Recidivism." *The Prison Journal* (March): 279–303.

Egan, Paul. 2015. "Michigan to End Prison Food Deal with Aramark." *Detroit Free Press,* 13 July. https://www.freep.com/story/news/local/michigan/2015/07/13/state-ends-prison-food-contract-aramark/30080211.

Fleetwood, Nicole R. 2020. *Marking Time: Art in the Age of Mass Incarceration.* Cambridge, MA: Harvard University Press.

Garcia-Vega, Ismael "Q." 2020. "A Citizen Without a Home." In *My Body Was Left on the Street: Music Education and Displacement,* edited by Kinh T. Vü and André de Quadros, 166–72. Boston: Brill.

Garrett, Burgess Wilson. 1908. *Marble Rock Journal* 5, 14 May.

"The GEO Group, Inc. Form 10-K for Fiscal Year Ended December 31, 2017." EDGAR. Securities and Exchange Commission, 20187, https://www.sec.gov/Archives/edgar/data/0000923796/000119312518058566/d494769d10k.htm

Gidda, Mirren. 2017. "Private Prison Company GEO Group Gave Generously to Trump and Now Has a Lucrative Contract." *Newsweek,* 11 May. https://www.newsweek.com/geo-group-private-prisons-immigration-detention-trump-596505.

Gilmore, Ruth Wilson. 2022. *Change Everything: Racial Capitalism and the Case for Abolition.* Chicago: Haymarket Books.

Ginsburg, Rebecca, ed. 2019. *Critical Perspectives on Teaching in Prison: Students and Instructors on Pedagogy behind the Wall.* New York: Routledge.

Glaze, Lauren, and Laura M. Maruschak. 2010. "Parents in Prison and Their Minor Children." *Bureau of Justice Statistics Special Report.* Washington,

DC: US Department of Justice Office of Justice Programs. https://bjs
.ojp.gov/content/pub/pdf/pptmc.pdf.

Gotsch, Kara. 2018. "Families and Mass Incarceration." Center for Advanced
Studies in Child Welfare (Spring), 7. https://cascw.umn.edu/
wp-content/uploads/2018/04/CW360_Spring2018_WebTemp.pdf.

Gurnon, Bill. 2018. *Three O' Clock Movement: Revelation in a Women's Prison*.
Prior Lake: The Story-Booker.

Haney, Craig. 2001. "From Prison to Home: The Effect of Incarceration and
Reentry on Children, Families, and Communities." Washington, DC:
US Department of Health and Human Services, December. https://aspe
.hhs.gov/basic-report/psychological-impact-incarceration-implications
-post-prison-adjustment#II.

Harry, Adam G., Mary L. Cohen, and Liz Hollingworth. Forthcoming. "An
Evaluation of a Musical Learning Exchange: A Case Study in a U.S.
Prison." *International Journal of Music Education*.

Hartnett, Stephen John, ed. 2011. *Challenging the Prison-Industrial Complex:
Activism, Arts, and Educational Alternatives*. Urbana: University of Illinois
Press.

Heitzig, Nancy A. 2016. *The School to Prison Pipeline: Education, Discipline, and
Racialized Double Standards*. Santa Barbara: Praeger.

Hendricks, Karin S. 2018. *Compassionate Music Teaching: A Framework for
Motivation and Engagement in the 21st Century*. Lanham: Rowman and
Littlefield.

Higgins, Lee. 2012. *Community Music in Theory and in Practice*. New York:
Oxford University Press.

Hinsley, Matthew, Travis Marcum, and Jeremy Osborne. 2016. "The Paper
Guitar: Changing Lives in the Guitar Classroom." *American String
Teacher* 66, no. 4: 36–37.

Hinton, Elizabeth. 2016. *From the War on Poverty to the War on Crime*.
Cambridge, MA: Harvard University Press.

Hodson, Raymond G. 1951. "A Survey of Music Education Programs in State
Prisons." MA thesis, University of Denver.

Horsley, Paul. 2006. "Prison-Based Singers Leave Sound Impression." *Kansas
City Star*, 20 January.

Howe, Emily, André de Quadros, Andrew Clark, and Kinh T. Vü. 2020. "The
Tuning of the Music Educator: A Pedagogy of the 'Common Good' for
the Twenty-First Century." In *Human Music Education for the Common*

Good, edited by Iris M. Yob and Estelle Jorgensen, 107–26. Bloomington: Indiana University Press.

Icenogle, Grace, Laurence Steinberg, Natasha Duell, Jason Chein, Lei Chang, Nandita Chaudhary, Laura Di Giunta, et al. 2019. "Adolescents' Cognitive Capacity Reaches Adult Levels Prior to Their Psychosocial Maturity: Evidence for a 'Maturity Gap' in a Multinational, Cross-Sectional Sample." *Law and Human Behavior* 43, no. 1: 69–85.

Johnson, Megan. 2007. "Coming Full Circle: The Use of Sentencing Circles as Federal Statutory Sentencing Reform for Native American Offenders." *Thomas Jefferson Law Review* 29, no. 2: 265–88.

JPI (Justice Policy Institute). 2011. "Finding direction: Expanding criminal justice options by considering policies of other nations." http://www .justicepolicy.org/uploads/justicepolicy/documents/sentencing.pdf.

Kaba, Mariame. 2021. *We Do This 'Til We Free Us: Abolitionist Organizing and Transforming Justice*. Chicago: Haymarket Books.

Kaplan, Ilana. 2020. "Record Label Die Jim Crow, Dedicated to Music by Prison Inmates, Is Toppling Stereotypes," *Los Angeles Times*, 26 June. https://www.latimes.com/entertainment-arts/music/story/2020-06-26/ die-jim-crow-record-label-prison-inmates.

Kaplan, Max. 1955. *Music in Recreation, Social Foundations and Practices.* Champaign: Stipes.

Kavanaugh, Lee H. 2006. "Choir Helps an Inmate Reconnect with His Family." *Kansas City Star*, January 22, A1, A13.

Kelley, Robin D.G. 2020. "Abolition then and now: Isaac Julien and Robin D.G. Kelley." Visualizing Abolition UC Santa Cruz Online Series, 1 December. https://ias.ucsc.edu/events/2021/abolition-then-and-now-isaac-julien-and-robin-dg-kelley-december-1-2020.

Kelly-McHale, Jacqueline. 2018. "Equity in Music Education: Exclusionary Practices in Music Education." *Music Educators Journal* 104, no. 3: 60–62.

King, Jr. Martin Luther. 1963. *Strength to Love*. New York: Walker and Company.

———. 1967. *Where Do We Go from Here: Chaos or Community*. New York: Harper and Row.

King, Stephen. 2000. *On Writing: A Memoir of the Craft*. New York: Charles Scribner's Sons.

Knopp, Fay Honey. 1991. "Community Solutions to Sexual Violence: Feminist/ Abolitionist Perspectives." In *Criminology as Peacemaking*, edited by

Harold E. Pepinsky and Richard Quinney, 181–193. Bloomington: Indiana University Press.

Knopp, Fay Honey, Barbara Boward, Mary Jo Brach, Scott Christianson, Mary Ann Largen, Julie Lewin, Janet Lugo, Mark Morris, and Wendy Newton. 1976. *Instead of Prisons: A Handbook for Abolitionists*. Syracuse: Prison Research Education Action Project.

Krinsky, Miriam, and Liz Komar. 2021. "'Victims' Rights' and Diversion: Furthering the Interests of Crime Survivors and the Community." *Southern Methodist Law Review* 74, no. 3: 527–44.

Ladson-Billings, Gloria. 1995. "Toward a Theory of Culturally Relevant Pedagogy." *American Educational Research Journal* 32, no. 3: 465–91.

———. 2014. "Culturally Relevant Pedagogy 2.0: a.k.a. The Remix." *Harvard Educational Review* 84, no. 1: 74–84.

———. 2017. "The (R)evolution Will Not Be Standardized: Teacher Education, Hip Hop Pedagogy, and Culturally Relevant Pedagogy 2.0." In *Culturally Sustaining Pedagogies: Teaching and Learning for Justice in a Changing World*, edited by Django Paris and H. Samy Alim, 141–56. New York: Teachers College Press.

Landreville, Donald J. 1956. "Comparative Study of the Uses of Music at the Montana State Prison with Prisons of the Northwest Area." MA thesis, Montana State University.

Le Mars Semi-Weekly Sentinel. 1909. "Music – The Second of Warden Sander's Reforms," 21 December, cols. 2–4.

Lederach, John Paul. 2005. *The Moral Imagination: The Art and Soul of Peacebuilding*. Oxford: Oxford University Press.

Lee, Oscar. 1924. *21st Biennial Report of the Wisconsin State Prison*, 30 June. Madison.

Lerman, Liz, and John Borstel. 2003. *Liz Lerman's Critical Response Process: A Method for Getting Useful Feedback on Anything from Dance to Dessert*. Takoma Park: Liz Lerman Dance Exchange.

Lieberman, Matthew. 2013. *Social: Why Our Brains Are Wired to Connect*. New York: Crown.

Liem, Marieke, and Nicholas J. Richardson. 2014. "The Role of Transformation Narratives in Desistance among Released Lifers." *Criminal Justice and Behavior* 14, no. 6: 692–712.

Liepmann, Moritz. 1928. "American Prisons and Reformatory Institutions: A Report." Translated [from German] by Charles. Fiertz. New York: National Committee for Mental Hygiene.

Lincoln NE *Star.* 1928 (30 November).

Lincoln Nebraska Evening Journal. 1924 (26 December).

———. 1929 (27 November).

Lincoln Nebraska Star. 1924 (23 December).

Littell, William J. 1961. "A Survey of the Uses of Music in Correctional Institutions in the United States." MA thesis, University of Kansas.

Love, Bettina L. 2020. "Abolitionist Teaching and the Future of Our Schools," 23 June. Featured video on the Abolitionist Teaching Network. https://abolitionistteachingnetwork.org.

Lozoff, Bo. 1985. *We're All Doing Time: A Guide to Getting Free.* Durham: Human Kindness Foundation.

Lucas, Ashley E. 2021. *Prison Theatre and the Global Crisis of Incarceration.* London: Methuen Drama, Bloomsbury.

Macy, Enceno. 2016. "Scarred by Solitary." In *Hell Is a Very Small Place: Voices from Solitary Confinement,* edited by Jean Casella, James Ridgeway, and Sarah Shourd, 121–24. New York: New Press.

Madden, Sidney, Sam Leeds, and Rodney Carmichael. 2020. "'I Want Us to Dream a Little Bigger': Noname and Mariame Kaba on Art and Abolition." NPR Music, "Louder than a Riot: Rhyme and Punishment in America." https://www.npr.org/2020/12/19/948005131/i-want-us-to-dream-a-little-bigger-noname-and-mariame-kaba-on-art-and-abolition.

Marcum, Travis. 2014. "Artistry in Lockdown: Transformative Music Experiences for Students in Juvenile Detention." *Music Educator Journal* (December): 32–36.

Martin, Buzzy. 2007. *Don't Shoot! I'm the Guitar Man.* New York: Penguin.

Maruna, Shadd. 2001. *Making Good: How Ex-Convicts Reform and Rebuild Their Lives.* Washington, DC: American Psychological Association Books.

———. 2011. "Reentry as a Rite of Passage." *Punishment and Society* 13, no. 1 (2011): 3–28.

———. 2017. "Desistance as a Social Movement." *Irish Probation Journal* 14 (2017): 5–20.

MATA (Music, Art, Theater Academy). n.d. "Voicing Transformation in Southwest Ohio Prisons" [newsletter].

Maycock, Matthew, and Kate Hunt, eds. 2019. *New Perspectives on Prison Masculinities.* Cham: Springer International.

McCarty, Teresa L., and Bryan McKinley Jones Brayboy. 2021. "Culturally Responsive, Sustaining, and Revitalizing Pedagogies: Perspectives from

Native American Education." *Education Forum* 85, no. 4 (2021): 429–43. doi:10.1080/00131725.2021.1957642.

McCoy, Kathleen. 2012. "'Jailhouse Bach' and Women of the Hiland Mountain Prison String Orchestra." *Alaska Public Media*, 23 November. http://www.alaskapublic.org/2012/11/23/jailhouse-bach-and-women-of-the-hiland-mountain-prison-string-orchestra.

McDaniels-Wilson, Cathy, and Joan Belknap. 2008. "The Extensive Sexual Violation and Sexual Abuse Histories of Incarcerated Women." *Violence against Women* 14, no. 10: 1090–127.

McNeill, Fergus. 2006. "A Desistance Paradigm for Offender Management." *Criminology and Criminal Justice* 6, no. 1: 39–62.

———. 2014. "Three Aspects of Desistance?" In *Discovering Desistance* (blog), An ESRC Knowledge Exchange Project, 23 May. https://discovering desistance.home.blog/2014/05/23/three-aspects-of-desistance.

Meiners, Erica R. 2011. "Ending the School-to-Prison Pipeline / Building Abolition Futures." *Urban Review* 43: 547–65.

———. 2016. *For the Children? Protecting Innocence in a Carceral State.* Minneapolis: University of Minnesota Press.

Meisenhelder, Thomas. 1982. "Becoming Normal: Certification as a Stage in Exiting from Crime." *Deviant Behavior* 3, no. 2 (1982): 137–53.

Méndez, Juan E. 2011. "Solitary Confinement Should Be Banned in Most Cases, UN Expert Says." *UN News*, 18 October. https://news.un.org/en/story/2011/10/392012-solitary-confinement-should-be-banned-most-cases-un-expert-says.

Messerschmidt, Edward. 2017. "Change Is Gonna Come: A Mixed Method's Examination of People's Attitudes toward Prisoners after Experiences with a Prison Choir." DMA diss., Boston University.

Mintz, Robert. 1974. "Interview with Ian Taylor, Paul Walton, and Jock Young." *Issues in Criminology* 9, no. 1: 33–53.

Montross, Christine. 2020. *Waiting for an Echo: The Madness of American Incarceration.* New York: Penguin Books.

Mullenbach, Cheryl. 2015 (27 January). "Prison warden with a heart," *Iowawatch.org.* https://www.iowawatch.org/2015/06/27/prison-warden-with-a-heart.

Murder Victims' Family for Human Rights. n.d. "Victims' stories: Renny Cushing. http://www.mvfhr.org/sites/default/files/pdf/gallery%20-%20cushing.pdf.

Murray, JaneAnne, Sean Hecker, Michael Skocpol, and Marissa Elkins. 2021. "Second look = Second chance: Turning the tide through NACDL's model second look legislation." National Association of Criminal Defense Lawyers. https://www.nacdl.org/Landing/Sentencing.

Nagin, Daniel S. 2013. "Deterrence in the Twenty-First Century." *Crime and Justice* 42: 199–263.

Nellis, Ashley. 2021. "No End in Sight: America's Enduring Reliance on Life Imprisonment." Washington, DC: The Sentencing Project. https://www.sentencingproject.org/publications/no-end-in-sight-americas-enduring-reliance-on-life-imprisonment.

Niccum, Jon. 2006 (20 January). "East Hill Singers Find Freedom through Song." *Lawrence Journal-World.*

OCC (Oakdale Community Choir). 2009. "IMCC-Community Choir Writing Sampler #1" [Newsletter], March. http://oakdalechoir.lib.uiowa.edu/2016/03/28/newsletter-march-2009/#more-5.

———. 2011. "Newsletter: May, 2011." http://oakdalechoir.lib.uiowa.edu/2011/05/01/newsletter-may-2011/#more-24.

Palidofsky, Meade, and Bradley C. Stolbach. 2012. "Dramatic Healing: The Evolution of a Trauma-informed Musical Theatre Program for Incarcerated Girls." *Journal of Child and Adolescent Trauma* 5, no. 3: 239–56.

Paris, Django, and H. Samy Alim. 2017. "What Is Culturally Sustaining Pedagogy and Why Does It Matter?" In *Culturally Sustaining Pedagogies: Teaching and Learning for Justice in a Changing World*, edited by Django Paris and H. Samy Alim, 1–24. New York: Teachers College Press.

Pepinsky, Hal. 2013. "Peacemaking Criminology." *Critical Criminology* 21: 319–39.

Perkins, Tom. 2018a. "Prison Guards: Michigan Is Deliberately Hiding Extent of Prison Kitchen Horror Show." *Detroit Metro Times*, 23 May. https://www.metrotimes.com/food-drink/prison-guards-michigan-is-deliberately-hiding-extent-of-prison-kitchen-horror-show-12271285.

———. 2018b. "We Spoke with Michigan Inmates about Rotten Food, Maggots, and More Kitchen Problems." *Detroit Metro Times*, 18 January. https://www.metrotimes.com/food-drink/we-spoke-with-michigan-inmates-about-rotten-food-maggots-and-more-prison-kitchen-problems-8686387.

Pfaff, John F. 2017. *Locked In: The True Causes of Mass Incarceration and How to Achieve Real Reform*. New York: Basic Books.

Prison Songs. 1997. "Historical Recordings from Parchman Farm 1947–1948: Volume One: Murderous Home." Rounder Records, CD.

"Prisoners Keep Time by Playing Band Music." 1984. *The Courier-Journal* [Louisville], 7 March.

Pyles, Loretta. 2018. *Healing Justice: Holistic Self-Care for Change Makers*. New York: Oxford University Press.

Raher, Stephen. 2016. "Paging Anti-Trust Lawyers: Prison Commissary Giants Prepare to Merge," 5 July. Prison Policy Initiative. https://www.prisonpolicy.org/blog/2016/07/05/commissary-merger.

———. 2018 (24 May). "The Company Store: A Deeper Look at Prison Commissaries." Prison Policy Initiative. https://www.prisonpolicy.org/reports/commissary.html.

Ranney, Dave. 2005. "Chained Melody: Inmate's Introspective Song Serves as Apology, Anthem," *Lawrence Journal-World*, May 9, 1A, 4A.

Regehr, Cheryl, Mary Carey, Shannon Wagner, Lynn E. Alden, Nicholas Buys, Wayne Corneil, Trina Fyfe, Alex Fraess-Phillips, Elyssa Krutop, Lynda R. Matthews, Christine Randall, Marc White, and Nichole White. 2019. "Prevalence of PTSD, Depression, and Anxiety Disorders in Correctional Officers: A Systematic Review." *Corrections* 6, no. 5 (2019): 1–13.

Richmiller, Mary G. 1992. "Study of the Residual Effects of Music Education Experiences of a Prison Choir, Twenty-Nine Years after Participation." MA thesis, Southeast Missouri State University.

Rideau, Wilbert. 2010. *In the Place of Justice: A Story of Punishment and Deliverance*. New York: Vintage Books.

Robertson, Eddie. 2015. Unpublished interview by Community Voices Producer for 91.3 WYSO Radio Station in Yellow Springs, Ohio, Steve McQueen.

Rocque, Michael. 2017. *Desistance from Crime: New Advances in Theory and Research*. London: Palgrave Macmillan.

Roma, Catherine. 2010. "Re-Sounding: Refuge and Reprise in a Prison Choral Community." *International Journal of Community Music* 3, no. 1 (2010): 91–102.

———. 2018. "I Am Because We Are: Building Choral Communities." *Choral Journal* 59, no. 3: 28.

Sabo, Don, Terry A. Kuper, and Willie James London, eds. 2001. *Prison Masculinities*. Philadelphia: Temple University Press.

Salvador, Karen, and Jacqueline Kelly-McHale. 2017. "Music Teacher Educator Perspectives on Social Justice." *Journal of Research in Music Education* 65, no. 1: 6–24.

Santos, Michael G. 2006. *Inside: Life Behind Bars in America.* New York: St Martin's Press.

Sawyer, Wendy. 2016. "Probation: The leading type of correctional control." https://www.prisonpolicy.org/graphs/Correctional_control_by_type_1975-2015.html.

Sawyer, Wendy, and Peter Wagner. 2020. "Mass incarceration: The whole pie 2020." https://www.prisonpolicy.org/reports/pie2020.html.

Schenwar, Maya, and Victoria Law. 2020. *Prison by Any Other Name: The Harmful Consequences of Popular Reforms.* New York: New Press.

Scudder, Kenyon J. 1968. *Prisoners Are People.* New York: Greenwood Press.

Sered, Danielle. 2019. *Until We Reckon: Violence, Incarceration, and a Road to Repair.* New York: New Press.

Seymour, Cynthia, and Creasie Finney Hairston, eds. 2001. *Children with Parents in Prison: Child Welfare Policy, Program, and Practice.* Washington, DC: Child Welfare League of America.

Shalev, Sharon. 2011. "Solitary Confinement and Supermax Prisons: A Human Rights and Ethical Analysis." *Journal of Forensic Psychology Practice* 11, nos. 2–3: 151–83.

Share Song. Create Magic. Capturing the Memories of the 2012 World Choir Games, World Choir Games. 2012. Cincinnati: Pediment.

Shaw, Julia. 2020. *Culturally Responsive Choral Music Education: What Teachers Can Learn from Nine Students' Experiences in Three Choirs.* New York: Routledge.

Shieh, Eric. 2010. "On Punishment and Music Education: Towards a Practice for Prisons and Schools." *International Journal of Community Music* 3, no. 1 (2010): 19–32.

Shourd, Sarah. 2016. "Preface: A Human Forever." In *Hell Is a Very Small Place: Voices from Solitary Confinement,* edited by Jean Casella, James Ridgeway, and Sarah Shourd, vii–xii. New York: New Press.

Shouse, Deborah. 2021. "Tuning in to Others: Jamey Aebersold's Jazz Ministry Fairly Sizzles with Zeal." *Unity Magazine,* March–April, 32–35.

Silber, Laya. 2005. "Bars behind Bars: The Impact of a Women's Prison Choir on Social Harmony." *Music Education Research* 7, no. 2: 251–71.

Small, Christopher. 1998. *Musicking: The Meanings of Performing and Listening.* Middletown: Wesleyan University Press.

Smit, Dirk van Zyl. 2007. "Handbook of Basic Principles and Promising Practices on Alternatives to Imprisonment." Vienna: UN Office on Drugs and Crime. https://www.unodc.org/pdf/criminal_justice/

Handbook_of_Basic_Principles_and_Promising_Practices_on_ Alternatives_to_Imprisonment.pdf.

Snare, Annika. 1975. "Dialogue with Nils Christie." *Issues in Criminology* 10, no. 2 (Spring): 35–47.

Solitary Watch. n.d. "FAQ." https://solitarywatch.org/facts/faq.

Southern Journey of Alan Lomax: Words, Photographs, and Music. 2013. Library of Congress in Association with W.W. Norton.

Sporny, Vetold W. 1941. "The Value of Music in Correctional Institutions." MA thesis, Duquesne University.

Stattman, Ed. 1982 (17 January). "Convicts Flock to Course on Music in State Prison; Teacher Says Music Helps Parolees Stay Out." United Press International. https://www.upi.com/Archives/1982/01/17/Convicts -flock-to-course-on-music-in-state-prisonnewlnteacher-says-music-helps -parolees-stay-out/8779380091600/

Stevenson, Bryan. 2014. *Just Mercy: A Story of Justice and Redemption.* New York: Random House.

Sturup-Toft, Sunita, Eamonn O'Moore, and Emma Plugge. 2018. "Looking behind the Bars: Emerging Health Issues for People in Prison." *British Medical Bulletin* 125, no. 1: 15–23.

Swanson, Rebecca D. and Mary L. Cohen. Forthcoming. "Music-making in Prisons and Schools: Dismantling Carceral Logics" in *Oxford Handbook of Care in Music Education,* edited by Karin S. Hendricks. Oxford University Press.

Taylor, Ian, and Laurence John Taylor, eds. 1972. *Politics and Deviance: Papers from the National Deviancy Conference.* Harmondsworth: Penguin.

Ternström, Sten. 1999. "Preferred Self to Other Ratios in Choral Singing." *Journal of the Acoustical Society of America* 105, no. 6: 3563–74.

Thompson, Jason D. 2016. "The Role of Rap Music Composition in the Experience of Incarceration for African American Youth." PhD diss., Northwestern University.

Tutu, Desmond Mpilo. 1999. *No Future without Forgiveness.* New York: Doubleday.

Tylek, Bianca, Connor McCleskey, and Robert Rose. 2020. "The prison industry: Mapping private sector players." *Worth Rises.* https:// worthrises.org/theprisonindustry2020.

Ubuntu Men's Chorus. 2015. "Begin to Love." Recorded December 2015, London Correctional Institution, CD.

UN General Assembly. 2015. Resolution 70/175. "United Nations Standard Minimum Rules for the Treatment of Prisoners," 17 December. https://undocs.org/A/RES/70/175.

US Bureau of Labor Statistics. 2020. "Occupational Employment and Wages, May 2020: 33-3012 Correctional Officers and Jailers." https://www.bls.gov/oes/current/oes333012.htm.

US Department of Justice. 2020. Bureau of Justice Statistics. Annual Survey of Jails in Indian Country. Inter-University Consortium for Political and Social Research, 20 October. https://doi.org/10.3886/ICPSR38112.v1.

van de Wall, Wilhem. 1924. *The Utilization of Music in Prisons and Mental Hospitals: Its Application in the Treatment and Care of the Morally and Mentally Afflicted.* New York: National Bureau for the Advancement of Music.

Wagner, Peter. 2015. "In Memory of Nils Christie, 1928–2015." Prison Policy Initiative, 9 June. https://www.prisonpolicy.org/blog/2015/06/09/nils-christie.

Walsh, Kelly, Jeanette Hussemann, Abigail Flynn, Jennifer Yahner, and Laura Golian. 2017. "Estimating the Prevalence of Wrongful Convictions." Washington, DC: US Department of Justice. https://www.ojp.gov/pdffiles1/nij/grants/251115.pdf.

Washington, Derrick. 2020. "Wandered to Find a Rhythm." In *My Body Was Left on the Street: Music Education and Displacement,* edited by Kinh T. Vü and André De Quadros, 288–97. Boston: Brill.

Waters, Ann W. 1997. "Conducting a Prison Chorus: An Interview with Elvera Voth." *Choral Journal* (August 1997): 17–21.

Weber, Amanda. 2018. "Choral Singing and Communal Mindset: A Program Evaluation of the Voices of Hope Women's Prison Choir." DMA diss., University of Minnesota.

Widra, Emily, and Tianna Herring. 2021. "States of Incarceration: The Global Context 2021." Prison Policy Initiative. https://www.prisonpolicy.org/global/2021.html.

Williams, Rachel Marie-Crane, ed. 2003. *Teaching Arts behind Bars.* Boston: Northeastern University Press.

Wilson, Catherine. 2013. "If You Listen, I'll Tell You How I Feel: Incarcerated Men Expressing Emotion." PhD diss., University of Iowa.

Wilson, Harry. 2014. "Turning Off the School-to-Prison Pipeline." *Reclaiming Children and Youth* 23, no. 1 (Spring): 49–53.

Wright, Emily M., Patricia Van Voorhis, Emily J. Salisbury, and Ashley Bauman. 2012. "Gender-Responsive Lessons Learned and Policy Implications for Women in Prison: A Review." *Criminal Justice and Behavior* 39, no. 12 (2012): 1612–32.

Wright, John Wesley. 2019. "Prisons and the Power of Performance: Reflections on Vocal Coaching for Men and Women behind Bars." *Journal of Singing* 75, no. 5 (May–June): 573–7.

Yazzie, Robert. 1994. "Life Comes from It: Navajo Justice Concepts." *New Mexico Law Review* 24, no. 175: 175–90. https://transformharm.org/wp-content/uploads/2018/12/Life-Comes-from-It_-Navajo-Justice-Concepts.pdf.

Zapotosky, Matt, and Chico Harlan. 2016. "Justice Department Says It Will End Use of Private Prisons." *Washington Post*, 18 August. https://www.washingtonpost.com/news/post-nation/wp/2016/08/18/justice-department-says-it-will-end-use-of-private-prisons/?noredirect=on.

Zehr, Howard. 2015. *The Little Book of Restorative Justice.* New York: Skyhorse.

INDEX